COMMUNITIES OF PRACTICE IN HEALTH AND SOCIAL CARE

For
Vikky, Nao and Alex
John
Michael
Joey, Mark, Bethan and Jonathan

– A real family of practice!

COMMUNITIES OF PRACTICE IN HEALTH AND SOCIAL CARE

Edited by

Andrée le May

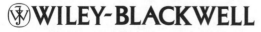

WILEY-BLACKWELL

A John Wiley & Sons, Ltd., Publication

This edition first published 2009
© 2009 by Blackwell Publishing Ltd

Blackwell Publishing was acquired by John Wiley & Sons in February 2007.
Blackwell's publishing programme has been merged with Wiley's global Scientific, Technical, and
Medical business to form Wiley-Blackwell.

Registered office
John Wiley & Sons Ltd, The Atrium, Southern Gate, Chichester, West Sussex,
PO19 8SQ, United Kingdom

Editorial offices
9600 Garsington Road, Oxford, OX4 2DQ, United Kingdom
350 Main Street, Malden, MA 021148-52020, USA

For details of our global editorial offices, for customer services and for information about how to
apply for permission to reuse the copyright material in this book, please see our website at
www.wiley.com/wiley-blackwell.

The right of the author to be identified as the author of this work has been asserted in accordance with
the Copyright, Designs and Patents Act 1988.

Library of Congress Cataloging-in-Publication Data

Communities of Practice in health and social care / edited by Andrée le May.
    p. ; cm.
  Includes bibliographical references and index.
  ISBN 978-1-4051-6830-4 (pbk. : alk. paper)   1. Communities of Practice.
2. Medicine—Practice.   3. Social service.   I. le May, Andrée.
  [DNLM: 1. Community Health Services.   2. Community Health Planning. WA 546.1 C7308 2009]

  R728.C58 2009
  362.12068—dc22

                               2008012705

A catalogue record for this book is available from the British Library

Set in 10/12.5pt Sabon by Aptara® Inc., New Delhi, India
Printed in Singapore by Markono Print Media Pte Ltd

1   2009

CONTENTS

FOREWORD

The health and social care field shows a growing awareness of the potential of Communities of Practice as an approach to learning, identity and innovation. Yet the relation of Communities of Practice and health and social care is a complex one. Communities of Practice are of course not new in health and social care. In fact, they are at its core. The history of health and social care is rooted in the formation of Communities of Practice – communities dedicated to learning how to care for patients with a discipline for optimal results. Indeed, the combination of a tradition of care for patients with a tradition of research and accumulated knowledge makes for a strong history of professional practice. It is as Communities of Practice that health and social care professions have earned the reputation of being able to address health and social issues – and the institutional legitimacy to do so.

This historical and social view of practice is reflected in learning processes for health and social care professionals. Whilst the field has accumulated a large body of theoretical knowledge, everyone knows that the actual practice cannot be fully learned in the classroom. Health and social care delivery remains a practice located in relationships, in interactions and in the improvisation inherent in situated intelligence. Therefore, in spite of the move into academic settings, there remains a strong tradition of practice-based learning, with extensive apprenticeship-like periods of internship.

There are therefore good reasons to focus on practice in health and social care today. The very definition of a professional is someone who can represent the best that a community has to offer in the provision of services. This makes active participation in relevant and productive Communities of Practice critical. The very publication of this book reflects a resurgence of interest in the learning that takes place in practice, both for the initial formation of health and social care professionals and for their continuing education as established professionals.

At the same time, an analysis of Communities of Practice on health and social care will reveal the ambivalence of their legacy. The institutionalisation of practice has given rise to very formalised communities that have accumulated power, access to training, titles and organisational structures. In health and social care as in other disciplines, Communities of Practice can be part of the problem as well as an opportunity for new learning. This is true not only in the context of health and social care delivery, but also in related contexts of research, management and policy-making. Indeed, professional knowledgeability in health and social care today depends on a constellation of interrelated practices. The health and social care industry constitutes a complex landscape of communities, both local and global, with distinct traditions, institutional formalisation, deep boundaries and established hierarchies. When practices form silos or fiefdoms, boundaries become static and create problematic disconnections.

Taking a Community of Practice perspective does not entail accepting existing practices and the way they are organised. On the contrary, a dynamic view of Communities of Practice highlights the possibility of finding learning partners independently of title or affiliation. The focus can be on learning what is necessary for the benefit of patients/clients. This is likely to give voice to new perspectives and invite new identities – both preconditions for reshaping the landscape. Progress in health and social care will require a lot of boundary crossing. For this, a focus on practice is a good way to start: caring for patients/clients in practice reflects the ethics of the profession and can create a motivating crucible for the renegotiation of boundaries.

Many of the Communities of Practice described in this book challenge the status quo and traditional boundaries. The function of Nurse Practitioner is a good example that combines traditional responsibilities of nurses and doctors. Working as a Community of Practice makes it much easier to go through such a substantial transition. It allows practitioners to develop their skills, build an identity and find a voice in their institutions.

Another challenging and challenged boundary is the relationship of patients with care-provider communities. The traditional view of the patient is a transactional role of receiving an expert service. Seeing the patient/client as a participant, even if peripheral, in health and social care, community is especially important today when everyone has multiple sources of knowledgeability about their conditions, including their own membership in Communities of Practice initiated and run by patients/clients. As patients, for instance, learning in such communities, they become increasingly active participants in the constellation of health and social care practices. It is therefore essential to include the patient's perspective explicitly into an account of social-learning processes in health and social care.

The book explores another important boundary where new Communities of Practice can make a substantial contribution – the north–south axis between the so-called developed and developing nations. The traditional perspective on this boundary is that knowledge flows from the north to the south. Working with Communities of Practice offers a different approach: rather than a simple transmission, the point is to create social containers for the negotiation of multiple perspectives into new practices. This makes for a very rich learning process – practices born of boundary encounters between medical science and perspectives on health from other cultures.

A social-practice perspective on health and social care is particularly relevant in today's complex health and social care systems, which tend to produce an increasing colonisation of practice by regulation and institutional prescription. This process reflects an inherent tension between the local, improvisational intelligence of practice and the need for standards, within institutions, and increasingly at a national and even global scale. A social-practice perspective allows us to value local practice without romanticising it and to value more systemic knowledge-production processes without denying local engagement its intelligence. Once we understand the knowledgeability of health and social care professionals as deriving from a whole landscape of practices, we can consider the learning dynamics that connect the whole system. From a community perspective, the learning potential of such a system lies in the combination of deep practices and active boundaries.

As key elements of these dynamics, Communities of Practice make it possible to give voice to new perspectives, to bridge boundaries between research and practice, to connect practitioners in new ways and to involve a broader range of stakeholders in addressing complex issues. To achieve their full potential, these emerging communities will have to combine local perspectives with systemic ones: the rigour of local intelligence with the rigour of cross-locality learning. It is in this tension between the local and the systemic that professionals make their most valuable and potentially creative contributions.

Books that start documenting these developments are welcome. We need cases and stories that illustrate the potential of Communities of Practice in health and social care without romanticising them. The realisation of this enormous potential will demand an acute awareness of the possibilities and pitfalls. Because of their self-organised nature, Communities of Practice can break free of established limitations; but for the same reason they can also, wittingly or unwittingly, reproduce patterns of dysfunction in their context. We need more books that approach the topic with an open yet critical mind. I hope this one is the beginning of a trend.

Etienne Wenger
North San Juan, California
March 2008

ACKNOWLEDGEMENTS

For Chapter 3

Linda would like to thank all the Nurse Practitioners in Interior Health who have not only made the CoP work but also helped her write this chapter by providing her with their thoughts. She would also like to extend her thanks to Tom Fulton for allowing her the autonomy to be both evidence informed, as well as creative, in the Nurse Practitioner integration plan.

For Chapters 4, 5 and 8

The authors of these chapters would like to thank the NHS Executive Office (South Thames) for funding these research projects, our co-workers Kathryn Edmunds, Harriet Jefferson, Robin Lovelock, Jackie Powell and Dale Webb and all who participated in the Communities of Practice we observed.

For Chapters 6 and 8

Andrée would like to thank John Gabbay and Jackie Powell, who were critical readers of these chapters (JG for 6; JP for 8).

For Chapter 9

Helen and Madeleine gratefully acknowledge ESRC funding on the What Works for Children project; all three authors acknowledge funding from the Nuffield Foundation on What Works, What Matters and What Counts: Preliminary Work on Cost-Effectiveness in Social Care with Children. Alan Shiell also gratefully acknowledges the financial support of the Alberta Heritage Foundation for Medical Research.

Helen Roberts and Alan Shiell are members of the CIHR-funded International Collaboration on Complex Interventions (ICCI). The ideas expressed in this chapter have benefited from discussion with our ICCI collaborators, and we gratefully acknowledge the financial support provided to ICCI by the Canadian Institutes of Health Research.

LIST OF CONTRIBUTORS

Mireille Brosseau is the programme officer for the Executive Training for Research Application (EXTRA) programme at the Canadian Health Services Research Foundation where she coordinates the curriculum and mentoring components of the programme. She also devotes some time to collaborating with colleagues on other Foundation initiatives such as Research Use Weeks and Community of Practice events.

Jane Coutts runs Coutts Communicates, a consulting firm specialising in writing, editing and knowledge transfer. Coutts Communicates works with national and provincial organisations and researchers, most, but not all, health-related. Jane also teaches plain-language writing and has given workshops at universities across Canada and in Australia.

John Gabbay is Emeritus Professor at the University of Southampton, where (1992–2004) he directed the Wessex Institute for Health R&D. Since qualifying in medicine at Manchester in 1974, he has mainly researched the social and organisational origins of medical knowledge, with a recent emphasis on the way knowledge enters practice.

Mary Gobbi is a Senior Lecturer in Nursing at the University of Southampton, where she is the research and evaluation lead for the Virtual Interactive Practice® initiative. Her clinical background is cardiothoracic and vascular nursing. She is also subject lead/co-coordinator for the nursing group in the EU Socrates Erasmus TUNING project which is developing pan-European competences for nursing graduates.

Judith Lathlean is Professor of Health Research, School of Nursing and Midwifery, University of Southampton, where she has been involved in projects using Communities of Practice to develop services. As an advocate of innovative research approaches that examine both processes and outcomes, she has also engaged in several action research studies in health and social care.

Alex le May works for Marie Stopes International supporting reproductive health programmes in Africa and Latin America and also studies at the London School of Hygiene and Tropical Medicine.

Andrée le May is Professor of Nursing at the University of Southampton, where she runs the Doctorate in Clinical Practice, and researches, teaches and writes about the use of knowledge in practice. She is particularly interested in Communities of Practice and how they promote knowledge sharing and encourage learning.

Michelle Myall is a Senior Research Associate in the Department of Primary Care and Population Science, University College London. Before that she was a Research Fellow at the School of Nursing and Midwifery, University of Southampton, where she worked on a Community of Practice project to develop outpatient services and other studies on new nursing roles.

Helen Roberts is Professor of Child Health at the Institute of Education, University of London. She is a member of the CIHR-funded collaboration on complex interventions, led from Calgary, and a member of the board of the National Institute for Health and Clinical Excellence (NICE).

Linda Sawchenko has worked in health care in British Columbia, Canada, in positions ranging from hospital administration to teaching and is an Adjunct Professor at the University of British Columbia, Okanagan. One of Linda's key responsibilities as Regional Practice Leader in Interior Health is the integration of Nurse Practitioners into communities in the interior of British Columbia.

Alan Shiell is Professor of Health Economics and member of the Population Health Intervention Research Centre at the University of Calgary. He holds a Health Scientist award from the Alberta Heritage Foundation for Medical Research and a CIHR Chair in the Economics of Public Health.

Madeleine Stevens is a Research Officer in the Social Science Research Unit at the Institute of Education, University of London. Her background is in research methodology and evidence-based policy and practice initiatives, including direct support to practitioners in social care.

Nina Stipich is the Director of the Executive Training for Research Application (EXTRA) programme. She joined the Canadian Health Services Research Foundation in March 2003 to lead the development and implementation of the newly announced EXTRA programme. She has worked in the research and science policy areas, ethics and international relations.

Part 1
INTRODUCING COMMUNITIES OF PRACTICE

The first part of this book introduces you to the concept of Communities of Practice and their relevance to health and social care.

Chapter 1

INTRODUCING COMMUNITIES OF PRACTICE

Andrée le May

Defining Communities of Practice

What are Communities of Practice (CoPs)? It would be difficult to improve upon Wenger *et al.*'s (2001: 4/5) description of them as:

> groups of people who share a concern, a set of problems, or a passion about a topic, and who deepen their understanding and knowledge of this area by interacting on an ongoing basis. ... These people don't necessarily work together on a day-to-day basis, but they get together because they find value in their interactions. As they spend time together, they typically share information, insight, and advice. They solve problems. They help each other. They discuss their situation, their aspirations, their needs. They think about common issues. They explore ideas and act as sounding boards to each other. They may create tools, standards, generic designs, manuals, and other documents; or they may just keep what they know as a tacit understanding they share. ... Over time, they develop a unique perspective on their topic as well as a body of common knowledge, practices, and approaches. They also develop personal relationships and established ways of interacting. They may even develop a common sense of identity. They become a community of practice.

This description immediately suggests why CoPs should be important for people who practice in health and social care settings. And indeed CoPs are increasingly forming, either naturally or through being deliberately created, as a mechanism for getting people together in order to develop best practice, implement new knowledge or shape old knowledge for new practices so that people might do their jobs better day to day. CoPs are ideal mechanisms through which people can discuss the best ways to implement knowledge to suit the needs and context of their area of practice or particular patients and therefore improve the quality of care that they give. CoPs can function either as real face-to-face communities or virtually via interactive learning environments or electronic discussion groups. To be effective, CoPs need to pay attention to the following (adapted from Lathlean & le May, 2002; Gabbay *et al.*, 2003):

- **Membership** in terms of choosing who is to be involved initially and throughout the life of the CoP, the extent (active or passive) and legitimacy of their involvement, their knowledge base and expertise, and the importance of their involvement to achieving the goal of the group and the alterations planned to care/services.
- **Commitment** from *within* the community to the desired goals and from *outside* the community in order to support any required service/practice alterations.
- **Relevance** to local communities and the existing services/professional groups/groups of patients to enable acceptance of the change.
- **Enthusiasm** that could be personal, professional or service related for the area being considered by the CoP.
- **Infrastructure** to support the work of the CoP in terms of ease of access to knowledge or evidence (e.g. availability of library resources and information technology, particular experts or opinion leaders) and resources which are available in order to find information about current services (e.g. networks, statistics and documents).
- **Skills** in relation to accessing and appraising a variety of sources of knowledge together with those needed in bringing evidence together into a coherent plan for action by the CoP. The latter, for instance, might involve writing action plans, reports or business plans.
- **Resources** for achieving the desired change that go beyond the time needed to meet, seek information or canvas support. These could include pump-priming money for pilot work in relation to the desired service change or funds for evaluating the effects of change on the quality of care provided by the new service.

Communities of Practice are beneficial not only for the people who form them, but also for the organisations within which, or across which, they function since they can be very powerful ways for sharing and applying knowledge whilst motivating participants to improve care. They therefore have the potential to positively impact on the:

- standard of care delivered to patients/clients;
- working environments and job satisfaction of the participants in the community;
- speed with which problems are solved;
- speed with which knowledge and innovation move into practice;
- creation of a unified team which may be uni- or multi-professional; and
- ownership and sustainability of changes to practice.

Furthermore, they can increase social, human, organisational, professional and patient capital – we will return to each of these as the chapter progresses.

Where did the idea of CoPs come from?

Although CoPs have existed for centuries, the term itself was coined only by Lave and Wenger in 1991 as a result of their analysis of apprenticeship learning in 'communities of practitioners' (Lave & Wenger, 1991: 29). Lave and Wenger's observations of apprentices showed learning to be a situated, social process dependent on, and developed through, interactions with others in their apprenticeship communities rather than the isolated, 'in the heads of individuals' (Hanks, 1991: 13) learning often assumed to exist in the classroom. The social learning experienced through the master–apprentice relationship, in which master and apprentice learned from and through each other, and the apprentices' interactions with each other and their wider community enabled successful learners to move from the edge (or 'periphery') of the community to full participation in its sociocultural practices. This is turn resulted in apprentices forming an identity with the community and then becoming new masters, or old-timers within the community, working with newcomers or their own apprentices, thereby rejuvenating the original CoP.

The essence, then, of a CoP seemed in this early work to be its potential for enabling learning to occur and knowledge to evolve through the social process of interacting with like-minded people – within and across CoPs – where the purpose of the interaction was directed by common activities/practice and knowledge exchange. Successful learning was characterised in a CoP not only by mastering skills and gaining knowledge but by becoming part of the community and as a result of that gaining a greater sense of identity as a participant in the community (Lave & Wenger, 1991: 111) and, one assumes, within the 'professional' group that the community reflected.

Wenger (1998) used this early work, together with his later observations of insurance claims workers, to formulate a conceptual framework – what he calls a social theory of learning – to explain how learning occurred in CoPs and as a result of this the purpose and functioning of CoPs. The theory of social learning, as described by Wenger (1998: 3), placed 'learning in the context of our lived experience of participation in the world', suggesting that it is 'a fundamentally social phenomenon' underpinned by four central premises:

1) We are social beings. ...
2) Knowledge is a matter of competence with respect to valued enterprises ...
3) Knowing is a matter of participating in the pursuit of such enterprises, that is, of active engagement in the world. ...
4) Meaning – our ability to experience the world and our engagement with it as meaningful – is ultimately what learning is to produce. (p. 4)

In addition, he set out an initial inventory of the components of the social theory of learning – meaning, practice, community and identity, all of which are integrated through the concept of the CoP. He defined each of these components as follows (Wenger, 1998: 5):

'*Meaning*: a way of talking about our (changing) ability – individually and collectively – to experience our life and the world as meaningful' (in terms of learning he refers to this as 'learning as experience').

'*Practice*: a way of talking about shared historical and social resources, frameworks, and perspectives that can sustain mutual engagement in action' (in terms of learning he refers to this as 'learning as doing').

'*Community*: a way of talking about the social configurations in which our enterprises are defined as worth pursuing and our participation is recognisable as competence' (in terms of learning he refers to this as 'learning as belonging').

'*Identity*: a way of talking about how learning changes who we are and creates personal histories of becoming in the context of our communities' (in terms of learning he refers to this as 'learning as becoming').

Meaning in CoPs is established, Wenger suggests, through an active process of participation, negotiation through continual interaction and the creation of artefacts (reification) that give form to this meaning (for instance, documents, guidelines for practice, protocols and directives as well as written descriptions of the workings of the CoP and its practice). This mutual engagement in the joint enterprise of the CoP also results in the creation of shared histories and identity stemming from a shared repertoire of practice, which in turn becomes a source of coherence for the community through which identity is created (and transformed) for both individuals and the community. A CoP is characterised by its collective pursuit of an enterprise/practice over a period of time in order to share significant learning and in some instances create new knowledge – 'learning is the engine of practice and practice is the history of that learning' (Wenger, 1998: 96).

So it seems safe to say that CoPs provide social infrastructures that foster learning. In order to achieve this, individuals, communities and organisations need to fulfil specific responsibilities towards learning – these include individuals engaging in, and contributing to, the practices of their communities and communities refining practice and regenerating their membership. Organisations hosting CoPs need to learn how to sustain these communities and enable links to develop between CoPs either within or outwith the organisation. Wenger (1998) suggests that this will occur through passing artefacts/documents/concepts (boundary objects) from one CoP to another, using the members themselves to broker elements of practice from one community into another often through conversations and meetings with, and making visits, to other CoPs (boundary encounters). These links will facilitate learning and the effective flow of knowledge across CoPs, and as a result organisations may better meet their goals and prosper whilst the CoPs remain hubs of learning.

These ideas are at the heart of Wenger's (1998) social theory of learning. He situates this theory at the centre of several polarised intellectual traditions reflecting theories of social structure and theories of situated experience, theories of practice and theories of identity, theories of collectivity and theories of subjectivity, as well as theories of power and theories of meaning. The complexity of this proposition, although never fully explained by Wenger, is reflected in Figure 1.1.

In the chapters that follow, it may be useful to use this framework to consider what the social structures of the CoPs are, how they direct (or not) the behaviour

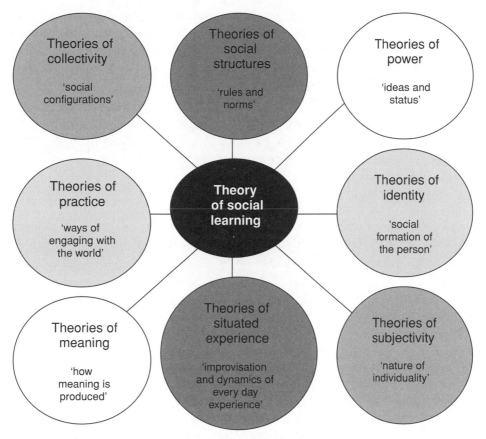

Figure 1.1 The conceptual underpinnings of Wenger's (1998) theory of social learning in Communities of Practice.

of the CoP's members, how power is played out in the CoPs, what meaning the CoP creates and what the CoP's collective function is. You might also consider how individuals, groups and organisations associated with the CoP benefit from its existence.

Designing for learning in CoPs

From what we know so far then it seems sensible to suggest that CoPs are useful structures through which learning, knowledge transfer, knowledge generation, problem solving, meaning and identity develop. If we accept their inherent and explicit value as a learning community, one of the questions that still remains to be answered is how – if learning, as suggested by Wenger (1998: 229) cannot be designed for, only facilitated or frustrated – can CoPs be designed in order to create favourable learning contexts? In other words, how can CoPs best be designed for learning?

In order to answer this, we need to work from the premise that the existence of a CoP alone does not make learning happen, just as the existence of a curriculum or classes or textbooks does not guarantee learning. CoPs are simply structures, albeit rather complex ones, that when at their most effective facilitate learning and when ineffective are likely to frustrate rather than effect learning. Wenger (1998: 229) describes CoPs as being about content:

> – about learning as a living experience of negotiating meaning – not about form. In this sense, they cannot be legislated into existence or defined by decree. They can be recognized, supported, encouraged and nurtured, but they are not reified, designable units. Practice itself is not amenable to design. In other words, one can articulate patterns or define procedures, but neither the patterns nor the procedures produce the practice as it unfolds. One can design systems of accountability and policies for Communities of Practice to live by, but one cannot design the practices that will emerge in response to such institutional systems. One can design roles, but one cannot design the identities that will be constructed through these roles.

There are certain things that can be done to encourage CoPs to develop – these have been detailed by Wenger *et al.* (2001) in their book *Cultivating Communities of Practice* and are further elaborated in the following chapters of this book. Whilst Wenger *et al.*'s proposals provide us with some design rules for the development and sustenance of CoPs, they also reflect the realisation that the CoP has the potential to 'steward knowledge inside organizations' (p. 220) and to extend knowledge systems 'beyond the boundaries of the firm' (p. 221), thus extending the impact of the CoP from one of learning and identity creation to one of enhancing organisational effectiveness and competitiveness and thereby increasing organisational capital.

In the first instance, a well-functioning CoP needs to develop and sustain three fundamental structural elements: domain, community and practice (Wenger *et al.*, 2001: 27–40). Without them it cannot function. The *domain* is the topic the community focuses on – it gives the members of the community a common ground to work with and provides a sense of identity thereby giving purpose to and generating value for the CoP's members and stakeholders. Having a clear domain also enables the CoP to interact with the organisation within which it is situated as well as other CoPs – they each have something to share, to develop, and to learn and to increase knowledge about. The *community* creates the 'social fabric of learning' (p. 28) within which the participants in the CoP are entwined. Working with the domain enables the community to determine and progress its common goals, which in turn generate trust and relationships between participants – these ensure that the CoP develops and is sustained. The *practice* is a set of frameworks, ideas, tools, language, stories and documents that the members of the community share – these represent the specific knowledge that the community develops, shares and maintains. This practice organises knowledge, tacit and explicit, codifiable and non-codifiable, in such a way that it represents the members' perspectives and allows knowledge to be transferred. However, these 'Communities of practice do not reduce knowledge to an object. They make it an integral part of their activities and interactions, and they serve as a living repository for that knowledge' (p. 9).

In addition to these three elements, Wenger *et al.* (2001: 51) highlighted seven design principles necessary for cultivating successful CoPs. These largely tell us not to stifle the evolving and dynamic nature of the CoP by over-directing its evolution but to create a vibrant environment through using both formal organised events or meetings and informal chats and exchanges to develop trust across its membership and stimulate ideas, which in turn are seeded beyond its boundaries through networking with others outside the CoP.

All CoPs go through a journey of development – this book tells the story of several CoPs in health and social care settings, each at a different stage of development and maturity. Even the most cursory reading of the stories conveys the key features of CoPs – domain, community and practice, as well as the learning that has occurred within them, or as a result of them, or still has the potential to occur. The case studies used in this book – which we hope will be capable of being translated into the reader's practice – show how CoPs develop social, human, organisational, professional and patient capital and as a result better patient/client care.

Communities of Practice – more than the social fabric of learning

Wenger's identification and discussion of the building blocks of social learning in CoPs provides us with a new vocabulary. Some might call it jargon! But it does give us the means to detail and explore the workings of CoPs – how they naturally develop, are sustained or closed; how we could manufacture or create such entities; how they impact on learning, on organisational effectiveness, on practice, on professional development and the development of professions; how and why they are used to transfer knowledge between people, communities and organisations. Briefly exploring these building blocks has allowed us, so far, to gain an understanding of how CoPs function as the 'social fabric of learning' (Wenger, 1996). We now need to move beyond this in order to expose their wider contribution to health and social care through the generation of social, human, organisational, professional and patient capital.

Using CoPs to generate social capital

For almost a century, scholars have been debating the ways in which concepts similar to social capital can be defined, used and measured, but the term, first used in the 1960s, has only more recently come into general use. Probably the best known and possibly the most contentious work in this field is Putnam's (2000) investigation of social change in North America and his resultant theory of 'social capital'. This theory defines social capital as 'the connections among individuals – social networks and the norms of reciprocity and trustworthiness that arise from them' (p. 19): these connections seem akin to those fostered between participants in CoPs and also between CoPs as they allow people to act together in order to effectively pursue shared objectives.

Putman describes social capital as having both individual and collective elements which benefit individuals, groups, organisations and society through encouraging citizens to resolve collective problems more easily, allowing communities to advance smoothly and extending awareness of the range of ways in which situations can be interpreted and dealt with. It is therefore not surprising that several writers (e.g. Lesser & Prusak, 1999; Daniel *et al.*, 2003) have linked CoPs with the creation of social capital, which in turn may be associated with organisational success. Organisations use CoPs' social capital to stimulate better knowledge management by, for example, enabling the quicker identification of experts or the more rapid brokering of agreements, thereby allowing knowledge to be found and used more efficiently and effectively by individuals, CoPs and organisations (Lesser & Prusak, 1999).

To gain the most from social capital, both the individual and the society (or the organisation) within which they function need to be well connected; this is true also for the CoP. For instance, when we think about social capital, Putnam (2000: 20) reminds us that 'A well-connected individual in a poorly connected society is not as productive as a well-connected individual in a well-connected society. And even a poorly connected individual may derive some of the spillover benefits from living in a well-connected community'. The same may be true for participants in a well or poorly connected Community of Practice. Putnam gives as an example of this the success of the IT industry in Silicon Valley in California when compared to a less successful IT community near Boston. The reason for the difference he suggests was nothing to do with expertise or resources; it was more strikingly to do with connections – personal relationships and networks in Putnam's terms – boundary working and the development of trust between (and within) CoPs in ours. The Boston community was deficient in these, whereas the Californian community was rich in them and prospered because of the free flows of information, mutual learning and reciprocity that occurred.

Thinking about the success of the Silicon Valley 'Communities of Practice' illustrates the relationship between, what Nahapiet and Ghoshal (1998) call, the three dimensions of social capital – structural, relational and cognitive – and CoPs. Successful CoPs provide participants with structural opportunities for networking within the CoP, between CoPs, from CoPs to the outside world and vice versa. In addition to these networking opportunities, successful CoPs act as a reference point for assessing members' knowledge without them having to go outside the CoP's boundaries; they also enable the initial assessment of new knowledge permeating the CoP to take place. Trust and respect are fostered by the CoPs ensuring that the relational aspect of social capital is maximised as too is the cognitive dimension not only through the knowledge generating and sharing nature of the CoP but also through the CoP's ability to create artefacts that can then be passed on and studied.

Generating social capital would appear to be one of the positive spin-offs of successful CoPs, and this in turn contributes to their ongoing success. However, it is not the generation of social capital alone that gives CoPs value in health and social care, it is also their capacity to merge social and human capital through learning that is important and in so doing generates organisational, professional and patient (or client) capital – all of which impact health and social care and the value that CoPs have in this arena.

Communities of Practice can generate human capital

Human capital is best described as the outcome of investment in people. This investment may take the form of, for instance, health or social care or, perhaps more conventionally and appropriately for us, the provision of education and/or training. Sharing knowledge and expertise in this way results not only in the possession of particular skills, dexterity (physical, intellectual, psychological, etc.) and judgement for the individual, but also in the facility to create outputs which may themselves be invested (Becker, 1964) in, for example, other people or organisations, thereby increasing 'capital' in some way.

Given this, it does not require too great a leap to recognise that the learning that occurs in a CoP generates human capital. For instance, in a CoP where newcomers learn from old-timers, the human capital of, for instance, the master (old-timer/expert) is invested in the development of the human capital of the apprentice (newcomer/novice); this knowledge sharing does not diminish the human capital of the master, it may even enhance it, but it does increase the human capital of the apprentice – and in doing so increases the collective human capital of the CoP. So participants in the CoPs learn from one another, CoPs learn from one another and in turn CoPs help to develop learning within organisations generating not only human capital but organisational capital too. There is a close relationship between human capital and organisational capital since the development and growth of organisations depends largely on the learning that occurs within them and the resultant return that they get from their investment in the people working in or involved with them.

Communities of Practice can generate organisational capital

Increasingly, CoPs are seen as mechanisms for transforming organisations through their contribution to the growth of organisational capital – 'the knowledge used to combine human skills and physical capital into systems for producing and delivering want-satisfying products' (Evenson & Westphal, 1995: 2237). Three broad components of organisational capital – workforce training, employee voice and work design (Black & Lynch, 2005) – would seem to be influenced by CoPs. CoPs enable effective knowledge transfer and learning, thereby affecting workforce training. Through participation they provide a voice for employees and influence workforce design by exposing knowledge, acting as a conduit for sharing it, solving problems and implementing change.

van Winkelen (2003) suggests that 'the driver for organizations to invest in developing CoPs is deeply rooted in their value as ways of transferring knowledge between people' and because of this they 'offer a form of social structure that can take responsibility for fostering learning, developing competencies and managing knowledge'. CoPs may therefore provide the vehicle through which knowledge and human skills are combined and in so doing create advantage for the organisation; their importance may revolve around their potential for forming and holding corporate memories, transferring best practices and acting as a focus for innovation (Alani et al., 2002). A good example of this is the transformation of the World Bank, a Washington, DC-based organisation centred on reducing poverty in some of the world's poorest countries, from a simple lending organisation to a knowledge-sharing organisation. This was primarily achieved through the introduction of CoPs and storytelling as ways of sharing knowledge both within the organisation and outside it (Denning, 2005b).

Significant organisational capital makes organisations more effective and efficient, which in turn has the potential to make them better places to work. Given this potential, it is hardly surprising that CoPs are being rapidly embraced by organisations and the business community; attention has extended beyond the early explorations of CoPs as communities of learning (Lave & Wenger, 1991) to focus on their value as a mechanism for effectively managing organisational knowledge (Cox, 2005) and thereby influencing organisational capital.

Communities of Practice can generate professional capital

Let us move back now to Lave and Wenger's (1991) early ideas. In their book *Situated Learning*, they hypothesise that 'learners inevitably participate in communities of practitioners and that the mastery of knowledge and skills requires newcomers to move toward full participation in the sociocultural practices of a community' (p. 29). These communities, where there is a professional remit, are vast repositories of professional knowledge and skills – what I shall call 'professional capital'. Members endow their knowledge and skills to others who may be newcomers or old-timers within the community; this in turn bolsters the community's knowledge assets and leads to further growth in the community's professional capital.

Professional capital is a complex entity comprising several interlinking parts. These include the following:

- The knowledge and skills that characterise the professional group. At first glance this seems straightforward enough; however, ownership of this portfolio is often unclear since, as in health and social care, it is frequently shared across professional groups.
- The sociocultural practices of the professional group.
- The formal and informal networks used to guide and develop practice.
- The written and unwritten rules that guide professional practice.

Professional capital is developed and amassed at several different levels of any profession; for instance, professional capital can reside in individuals, in educational and/or research establishments, in the literature, in CoPs (one person may belong to many) or in the profession's governing/guiding bodies (for instance, Royal colleges, professional and statutory bodies, professional associations/societies). Professional capital may be variously viewed across and between professions. For instance, sub-groups within a profession may distinguish between different groups' professional capital by assigning greater or lesser respect to it – this may also happen between professions (Chau, 2005) and in turn lead to competition or distrust rather than collaboration between groups and professions with a resultant undermining of professional capital.

It is relatively easy to extrapolate Lave and Wenger's (1991) observations of learning in CoPs to the health and social care arena and the acquisition and growth of professional capital. New students start their studies on the edge of a community of knowledgeable and skilled practitioners moving, as they master essentials of the repository of professional capital, closer to full participation. Mary Gobbi describes this process for nurses in Chapter 6. Having passed through their 'apprenticeship' to full participation, or from being a novice to an expert practitioner, they continue to contribute to the wealth of that community whilst belonging to other specialist/role-related CoPs. Whilst these specialist/role-related CoPs work towards fine-tuning practices and solving problems, they continue to shape the sociocultural practices of the profession. Sometimes the professional capital generated by these CoPs is reified and made explicit for reinvestment – sometimes reinvestment occurs more randomly, experientially through role modelling, listening and watching as practice unfolds. Chapter 5 written by John Gabbay and me gives a sense of the way in which Communities of Practice can contribute to and influence the continuous development of professional capital for doctors working in primary health care.

Communities of Practice can generate patient capital

Just as CoPs can generate professional capital, they can generate what I shall call patient (or client) capital. In fact within the broad landscape of health and social care, one cannot exist without the other – professional capital and patient capital are interdependent and mutually constituted. Wenger (1998: 6/7) reminds us that CoPs 'are everywhere', that they are 'an integral part of daily lives' and as such have for centuries provided a 'non-professional' social fabric for learning. Why then not take this one step further and think about how CoPs populated by patients or their representatives might generate patient capital?

Patient capital, whilst encompassing human capital, is the product of a distinct learning experience – one focused on health and social care through the lens of the recipient. This type of capital accumulates by learning from, for instance, the way people view their health and social situation, their satisfaction with health and/or social care services, their expectations of care and their plans for being involved in, or changing, that experience. Generating and exposing this capital in CoPs builds a store that can then be used not only by others with similar experiences but also by professional caregivers, so also contributing to the stocks of professional capital. This process arguably has the potential to transform problems experienced individually into public issues (Gibson, 2006).

The potential to generate patient capital through CoPs is manifested in two ways. The first is through the involvement of patients or people who represent their views in multi-agency, multi-professional CoPs (Gabbay *et al.*, 2003). In order for this to be a success, patients need to use strategies that make this type of capital explicit and communicate it effectively so that rather than sinking without trace in an assertive articulation of professional capital, it contributes to and advances it. I explore this a little more in Chapter 8 by considering how storytelling has been used in such CoPs to articulate the patient/client/lay voice and thus generate patient capital, which in turn advances care (not least by helping to improve professional capital). Secondly, patients can establish CoPs in order to explore a domain of health and social care perhaps originally through support groups or patient/client representative groups. The patient capital generated by these CoPs does not immediately have to compete with professional capital – rather this is done once the CoP exposes its work to others. Although it is not dealt with in this book, there may be merit in considering the role of patient organisations as a vehicle for enhancing patient capital through CoPs.

Whilst you are reading the case studies in the following chapters and thinking about the different sorts of capital that they may generate, it might be useful to think about what belonging to a CoP does for individuals, for the CoP collectively, for the organisation in which the CoP is situated and also for the professional or patient/client group that the CoP is situated in.

What can go wrong?

So far CoPs have been portrayed in a positive light, offering benefits for individuals, teams, organisations and professional or patient communities as the CoP's knowledge is moved into the wider community within which, for us, care is provided. However, Wenger *et al.* (2001) warn that CoPs can also have their dark side, which rather than enabling learning stifles it.

There are a variety of ways in which the CoP can go wrong – some develop from within the CoP, others have their origins outside the CoP. Things tend to go wrong within the CoP either at a structural level or at an individual level. At the structural level failings might occur, perhaps as a result of the CoP being unable to fulfil all the criteria for successful working detailed above or not having a consistent membership; at the individual level, problems might occur as a result of some members becoming, for instance, too possessive of knowledge, believing the CoP to have a monopoly on that knowledge and ultimately resisting its transfer beyond the boundaries of the CoP (Brown & Duguid, 2001). Individuals may also form cliques within the CoP which hinder learning and knowledge transfer within it and smother participation. Or it might be that the CoP fails to link up with others or cannot find new members; its members become mistrustful of each other or it is unsupported or overly controlled (Thompson, 2005) by its organisation because of internal politics or irrational fears of the CoP becoming too strong to contain – all of these will cause the CoP to perish.

Ardichvili *et al.* (2003) found knowledge hoarding in virtual Communities of Practice to be a problem. However, this was not knowledge hoarding for selfish reasons associated with power or status, it was knowledge being hoarded primarily because people were afraid to share it – either because of their fear of providing the wrong information, being criticised or having their knowledge belittled by others, or because they were uncertain as to whether or not their position in the organisation was high enough for their knowledge to be of any use. To counter this problem, they advocate face-to-face communities where participants get to know and trust each other more quickly than in virtual communities and also remind readers of the need to have supportive organisational structures which encourage and nurture CoPs rather than manage and stifle them leaving little room for creativity and learning.

Why are CoPs important?

As I have already suggested, Communities of Practice are different from other groups usually found in organisations providing health and social care in that they are first and foremost learning communities and as such we should be able to tell them apart from others. As a learning community their purpose is to develop members' capabilities by building and exchanging knowledge (van Winkelen, 2003) within the CoP and the organisation, rather than achieving a task or delivering a product/service as is the case with working or project groups. The learning that accompanies this process requires the CoP to be adaptable and open to change, which in turn enhances the CoPs usefulness to the organisation by making it better able to adapt organisational processes to suit client needs. This is particularly important in organisations providing health and social care since the dynamic and flexible nature of the CoP suits the dynamic and flexible needs of the varied groups that either use or work in these organisations. In turn, health and social care organisations benefit from CoPs' potential to integrate learning into practice and to generate learning from the discussion of practice experiences. Chapter 5 describes how this happens in primary health care, whereas in Chapter 7, Alex le May describes how CoPs can be used more widely to develop health care across global boundaries.

Communities of Practice are often described as places for developing new practices, new services and new products (Coakes & Smith, 2006). Nina Stipich, Jane Coutts and Mireille Brosseau in Chapter 2 write about the experiences of the first 'graduates' from the EXTRA (Executive Training for Research Application) programme in Canada as they sought to improve health and social care by promoting research-informed management in Canadian health care organisations. They have supported each other in this endeavour by forming a Community of Practice. In addition to this, Linda Sawchenko in Chapter 3 tells the story of how

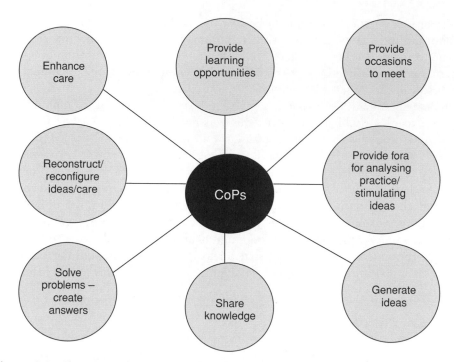

Figure 1.2 The potential of Communities of Practice in health and social care.

a CoP developed in British Columbia to support Nurse Practitioners and how they not only enhanced their own knowledge and confidence through the CoP but also transferred this knowledge to their practice and improved patient care. Judith Lathlean and Michelle Myall in Chapter 4 describe how one 'constructed' Community of Practice developed learning around dermatology practices and transferred their learning to the wider health and social care world through an interactive database.

In an increasingly time-pressured and competitive world, CoPs provide opportunities for enhancing the effectiveness and efficiency of our practice as well as generating social, human, organisational, professional and patient capital. Their dynamic nature affords them multiple opportunities for creating learning and developing care through analysis, creative thinking and the sharing of ideas (see Figure 1.2).

But as we have seen, there are limitations and potential problems. We therefore need to know how effective they are in health and social care – later in this book (Chapter 9) Helen Roberts, Alan Shiell and Madeleine Stevens provide us with some ways for looking at this. Part of maximising the potential of CoPs to enhance services is to learn from, and evaluate, the experience of using them. It is hoped that the case studies presented here will allow us to begin that process.

Part 2
GETTING STARTED

In the second part of this book, Nina Stipich, Jane Coutts and Mireille Brosseau; Linda Sawchenko; Judith Lathlean and Michelle Myall tell their stories about starting Communities of Practice. They have very different experiences and aspirations for each of the three Communities of Practice (CoPs). In Chapter 2, Nina, Jane and Mireille tell the story of the EXTRA CoP. A CoP constructed purposefully by the Canadian Health Services Research Foundation (CHSRF) in order to facilitate better, research-informed, decision making by health service managers and policy-makers across the Canadian health care system. Nina, Jane and Mireille tell the story of the beginnings of this CoP and how the CHSRF engineered it into existence.

Linda's story on the other hand relates to a more local initiative helping newly recruited Nurse Practitioners to integrate into a western Canadian Health Authority through the development of a Community of Practice. This CoP has been running now for some time and her account in Chapter 3 of the participants' experiences and their colleagues' views of them clearly shows how a CoP, albeit a constructed rather than a naturally occurring one, can help to form identity, develop and articulate practice and become a means for raising the profile of a particular professional grouping within health and social care.

Both of these Communities of Practice, if successful, clearly have the potential to increase social, human, organisational and professional capital within the health and social care arena.

In Chapter 4, Judith and Michelle tell a somewhat different story of CoP development in dermatology outpatient services. Their honest appraisal of the process and outcome of facilitating a CoP into existence exposes the tense relationships that can form in and around CoPs and how, despite these, successful outcomes might be achieved.

Chapter 2

THE EXTRA COMMUNITY OF PRACTICE: INCUBATING CHANGE

Nina Stipich, Jane Coutts and Mireille Brosseau

Introduction

The EXTRA programme – Executive Training for Research Application – trains health system managers and policy-makers how to use research in decision making. And then it sets them on a course to become a Community of Practice, supporting and reinforcing each other's efforts to promote the use of research in delivering health services. To make the transformation from a community of learners to a Community of Practice, EXTRA graduates must create a domain of shared interests that will let them function as something more than a network or an alumni group. They need to draw on resources and networks beyond their own membership, foster sub-communities around shared interests and regional issues and find the resources to sustain the new community, including annual face-to-face events, technological infrastructure and dedicated leadership. This chapter traces that journey.

From conception to realisation

The Executive Training for Research Application (EXTRA) programme takes accomplished health care leaders at the height of their careers and turns them back into students in a 2-year programme to develop the skills and knowledge to find, adapt and use research to run their organisations better. But the EXTRA fellows are a hybrid kind of student, who balance 3 weeks a year of classroom time with 49 weeks of applying their theory to the real-world problems of the organisations they work for.

EXTRA is the most ambitious effort so far of the Canadian Health Services Research Foundation (CHSRF, 2003a, 2007) to promote research use in health services. CHSRF was created in 1997 in recognition that the capacity to produce good and relevant health services research was important to the quality and sustainability of the country's health care system. From the beginning, the Foundation has focused on 'linkage and exchange', encouraging researchers, policy-makers and decision makers to work together on health services research (Lomas, 2000). But over the years, a further need, to increase the ability of health care decision makers to understand research and to apply it in their organisations, emerged (CHSRF, 2003b). That was the origin of EXTRA.

The goals of EXTRA are not confined to its formal 2-year span. It was always the plan that EXTRA graduates would evolve from an organised learning community into a Community of Practice. When members join EXTRA's Community of Practice, they have 2 years of building relationships behind them, advanced technology at their fingertips to link them to research and each other, and staff and budget dedicated to promoting continued learning. This commitment to continue arises from the belief that use of evidence in health services delivery will gain acceptance more widely and quickly through a Community of Practice than through EXTRA graduates alone spreading the word.

As it happened, the first cohort of EXTRA fellows was not even close to graduating when two of them, Vincent Tam and Denise Mauger, both executives from rehabilitation centres in Montreal, found themselves working together to apply their training in evidence use to the merger of their organisations. Mergers (proposed and real) of health organisations have dominated Canadian health care for the past 15 years. Too often, however, the shape of the new organisations has been determined by a mix of turf wars, tradition and expediency. Tam and Mauger wanted to do what they could to ensure decisions about the merger were based on solid research evidence. They decided to work together to help design the merged organisation based on what research showed was the best model for the most effective care. After consulting with clinicians, they searched out evidence on the ideas and recommendations they had gathered.

Without their collaboration, the result would have been very different from what had been planned, says Tam, director of rehabilitation services at the Lindsay Rehabilitation Hospital. 'People internally were pushing to expand the scope, to try to be everything to everyone, but the literature says you cannot develop expertise when you diversify that much', he says. Research clearly showed, for example, that a proposal the Lindsay's services be extended to cancer patients would not have been a good use of its highly intensive style of rehabilitation; cancer patients need a slower-paced, less-intensive model.

Similarly, with most staff focusing on how to get resources to preserve the status quo, Tam and Mauger, director of organisational development at the Institut de réadaptation de Montréal, looked for research on what resources a merged rehabilitation centre would need to give optimal care to the appropriate clients. 'EXTRA allowed us to be conscious of the reasons we proposed the things we did and to question ideas and objectives', Tam says.

The fact Tam and Mauger were starting to operate as a Community of Practice even before their 2-year programme was finished is good news for the CHSRF, which operates EXTRA on behalf of a consortium of partners. The Foundation's hope is that by the end of EXTRA's planned 10-year lifespan, it will have proved to be the catalyst of a national community of health care executives who encourage and oversee the use of research evidence in all decisions at their organisations and health regions. Two EXTRA fellows spontaneously deciding to pool their knowledge and resources suggests that the plan for a well-supported Community of Practice should work.

The catalyst

Since its creation, CHSRF has made the concept of knowledge transfer an integral part of health services research. It has put equal emphasis on promoting *exchange*, the crucial researcher–decision maker interactions that allow knowledge to be transferred, ensuring research reflects the reality of administering and delivering health care. But whilst the theory of knowledge transfer and exchange was developed and refined, there was not a programme to promote research literacy and develop a culture of evidence-based decision making in the health care system. Three national organisations – the Canadian Medical Association, the Canadian Nurses Association and the Canadian College of Health Services Executives – joined the CHSRF to discuss goals for such a programme and to define its focus (CHSRF, CAN, CCHSE, le Consortium quebecios, and CMA, 2004). They agreed to create the Executive Training for Research Application programme. It became a reality quickly after the federal government agreed to support the proposal. Canada gave the Foundation $25 million in 2003 to operate EXTRA for 10 years; the first cohort of 2 dozen executives began the programme the next year (Health Canada and CHSRF, 2003).

To be eligible, EXTRA applicants must be mid-career health service executives in senior positions, such as chief executive officer or chief of nursing or medicine. There are four residency sessions over the 2 years, covering topics from enhancing the fellows' own research literacy to showing them how to promote research use and develop the leadership skills they need to change their organisations. Throughout the programme, the fellows work on intervention projects in their home organisations, using research evidence to tackle a significant policy, programme or administrative issue. The intervention projects also play a part in laying the foundation for a Community of Practice. Fellows develop their projects working with mentors – experts in some aspect of health care relevant to the topic – through the Foundation's four regional mentoring centres (Atlantic Canada, Ontario, Quebec and Western Canada).

The partners behind EXTRA also include a consortium of 12 partners in Quebec, represented by the Agence des technologies et des modes d'intervention en santé, so there is always a good mix of fellows from a variety of organisations and health regions. The partners' goals were to hasten the cultural shifts needed to make the use of research evidence standard in health care decision making, support mentoring and promote collaboration among health service executives, nurses, physicians and researchers in the management of the health system. Overarching all was the desire to create a critical mass of health executives committed to research use, to speed up integration of research into every level of decision making in health care. Starting in 2007, this has been taken a step further by admitting teams of fellows from some organisations to let them build capacity for research use more quickly and thoroughly.

Fellows tend to leave their credentials behind when they enter the programme and much of the baggage of inter-professional rivalries as well. Members of the first group of fellows remember that about halfway through their first week of residency; there was an effort to organise them by profession for an exercise. Surprised and pleased at how completely they had ignored among themselves who was a physician, a nurse or some other kind of executive, they rejected the plan, sticking with their profession-free relationship.

Canada's English and French bilingualism can add considerably to the cost and complication of running a truly national programme, but all the partners agreed from the beginning that EXTRA could not be less than completely bilingual. The commitment to bilingualism is working very well – a third of participants come from Quebec. All meetings have simultaneous translation, although for practicality's sake, smaller workgroups are usually – but not always – divided by language. Free flow of ideas can be limited by the divide because people tend to socialise and network in their own language. That is likely to be a continuing challenge in the Community of Practice, of which more later.

The Foundation, however, is not content merely to train executives in research use and send them back to run their own organisations more efficiently and effectively. It wants to promote evidence use nationally and increase EXTRA's impact by keeping the fellows working together after the formal programme ends. The Foundation's goal is to create what Etienne Wenger and Jean Lave were the first to call a Community of Practice (Wenger, 2007) – a group of people who share a concern or a passion for something they do and learn how to do it better as they interact regularly.

According to Lave and Wenger (Wenger, 2007), a group must have a domain of shared interest, be a community and be practitioners to qualify as something more than a network or a community of interest. EXTRA fellows have the required *domain* of shared interest in their commitment to base health care decisions on research evidence. They become a *community* through two residency sessions a year (2 weeks in the summer and one in the winter, held in rural resorts where distractions are at a minimum). In the sessions, they engage in joint activities and discussions, help each other and share information and build relationships that enable them to learn from each other. Most fellows say they felt part of the group within the first few days, if not hours, of the programme. The fellows also definitely meet the requirement of being *practitioners*; in between sessions, they return to their demanding professional roles.

The 2-year, staggered-entry programme also lets the groups overlap allowing for networking and knowledge exchange. EXTRA alumni are already serving as mentors for new fellows entering the programme. The annual 2-week August residency session is a lively one, where three cohorts of EXTRA fellows overlap. New participants start the first two curriculum modules and begin to design their intervention projects. The cohort that is midway in the 2-year fellowship works on curriculum modules 4 and 5 and develops implementation plans for their intervention projects; they are joined by the cohort that has just finished the programme, there for a graduation ceremony and to start building the Community of Practice with their peers. About 150 health care executives, programme faculty and guests from across the country participate in the summer sessions. This annual event is an important catalyst for developing a long-term community.

Support for sustained learning and exchange

However, the Foundation is not inclined to leave the success of the EXTRA Community of Practice solely to occasional meetings or individual commitment and supports both the concept and reality of the community in many ways. During the programme and after graduation, fellows are invited to participate in events around the country organised or supported by the Foundation and EXTRA partners to keep them involved and in touch. The Foundation hosted events for EXTRA graduates at its national conferences in 2006 and 2007 for which the EXTRA Community of Practice steering group developed sessions and panels and brought in Canadian and international speakers.

EXTRA fellows are also invited to participate if one of the Foundation's Research Use Weeks is being held in their part of the country. Content in the sessions is tailored to each region and participants – health system managers and policy-makers – are introduced to an assortment of tools for using research (such as CHSRF's Self Assessment Tool, which measures an organisation's capacity to use research, inventories of promising organisational strategies for using research and the Researcher-Decision Maker Resource Guide). Research Use Weeks let members of the EXTRA Community of Practice hold sessions on strategies to improve organisational research use based on their intervention projects and lessons from the EXTRA programme.

The regional mentoring centres and partners also provide opportunities for EXTRA fellows to promote research use in their regions. In November 2007, the Quebec consortium of EXTRA partners organised a gathering for fellows, mentors and representatives of the partners, both to celebrate the graduation of the first group of fellows and to develop recommendations for sustaining and transferring the knowledge from the EXTRA programme. Participants, including 15 fellows from three cohorts, suggested strategies to ensure use of research-based evidence is build into organisational decision-making processes. By engaging the broader EXTRA community in advancing the use of research, the event also showed how the concept of a Community of Practice is not limited to being a post-programme entity.

Beyond face-to-face meetings, the prime tool for building the community and keeping it together is the EXTRA desktop. The desktop is a shared database designed for EXTRA and supported by the Centre for Health Evidence at the University of Alberta. Perceptions of how user-friendly it is vary, but all the fellows agree that the desktop's most important feature is its virtual library, which gives them access to 500 journals, databases (including the Cochrane Library, OVID Reviews, Catalogues et

Index des Sites Médicaux Francophones, PubMed, ABI Inform and more), sections on nursing policy, practice guidelines, news and other information.

Two tabs on the desktop – community and learning – comprise all the content from the residency sessions, information on Communities of Practice, support for the intervention projects and multiple tools to help fellows connect and work together, from bulletin boards to a common workspace that lets fellows share information – presentations, documents, files, records – and links to useful sites.

The desktop has another function, at least as important as its application during the EXTRA programme, according to Hayward. He is the Assistant Dean of Health Informatics and Director of the Centre for Health Evidence at the University of Alberta, which provides the technical support for the desktop. Hayward teaches the health information management curriculum for the EXTRA programme and he believes the desktop is crucial for keeping fellows engaged in a Community of Practice. 'To attract people to a Community of Practice, you have to give them something special', he says. Part of that is access to an 'incredible community of people' but to keep fellows coming back, Hayward says, 'we have to constantly refresh the stream of goodies. The desktop has to be the definitively best way to see what's new on the web.... They will just have more and more demands on their time, so it will have to be pretty amazing to bring them back'.

The foundation of the Community of Practice is laid out in the final weeklong residency module of the EXTRA programme. In the mornings, fellows present their intervention projects (the evidence-based change projects they have planned and implemented in their home organisations, which cover issues such as patient safety, recruitment and retention plans for physicians and nurses, and technology assessment). The afternoons are divided between learning new web and desktop skills useful for a Community of Practice, examining Community of Practice theory and deciding what they want from – and can give to – a Community of Practice. In 2007, the Foundation added something new to the final week – a special forum for CEOs where they were asked to identify themes to help shape the EXTRA programme. The Foundation also wanted to seed the creation of a network to help address necessary changes in Canadian health care – which worked so well, its looking for ways to link this new network to future Community of Practice initiatives. (There are other changes in the works for the final residency week. Future fellows will have read about Community of Practice theory before the session, so the face-to-face work can focus on developing knowledge transfer and exchange skills, such as using stories and anecdotes to promote evidence-informed decision making.)

Etienne Wenger led Community of Practice discussions for the first two cohorts, telling the fellows the reasons for joining a Community of Practice – these included helping each other solve problems, avoiding 'local blindness' and opening up the imagination, keeping up with change, reflecting on and improving practice and finding a common voice to gain influence. They occur naturally, but they can be seeded – and within them, it is what he calls 'social artists' that make them work, creating the connections that allow others to come along and learn. It takes work to sustain a Community of Practice; external supports help tremendously but dedication of members is just as important. 'You have to have members who care enough to do what it takes to nurture it', Wenger says.

Wenger tells the fellows that communities are difficult to sustain, partly because sentiment is not a real basis for a Community of Practice and partly because they must give good value for the time they take. 'Everyone says let's keep in touch, but unless it's useful to you in your daily life, it's not going to be sustainable (Wenger)'. Health care executives are tremendously busy people; most fellows agree that freeing up the time for EXTRA (both for the residency sessions and for their projects) has been very difficult; many admit to doubts they can keep up involvement beyond the commitment of the formal programme. If they do, they say, it is more likely to be sub-communities of practice, where fellows who have worked on quality, patient safety, or human resources will naturally turn to others facing the same types of issues. Reaching out to the broader community seems less likely.

Most fellows think, however, that face-to-face meetings will remain important. Canada's size has some fellows picturing regional groups: fellows in the Atlantic provinces or British Columbia could get together with each other more easily than whole cohorts can be brought to one place at one time. Few believe that there will ever be full participation in a Community of Practice, and there is a general feeling that Community of Practice meetings should be linked to other events fellows would attend anyway. Many of the CHSRF's partners in EXTRA (such as the Canadian College of Health Service Executives) hold national meetings that could add features to bring EXTRA fellows together.

Looking for direction

Doubts aside, the fellows value their EXTRA experience and would like to see a Community of Practice succeed. A steering committee of Cohort 1 fellows wrote terms of reference for a community, planning to focus on topics relevant to health care managers. Maureen Cava, manager of professional practice, planning and policy for Toronto's Department of Public Health, is on the steering committee. She says that they started by asking themselves what glue held the group together. The intervention projects can mostly be sorted into some broad categories, but looking further into some of those areas did not seem a sufficient bond for a Community of Practice. In the end they decided that 'excellence in leadership to promote evidence-informed decision making in health care organizations' was a common area of interest that could keep people engaged.

Steven Soroka, a fellow from Capital District Health Authority in Halifax, developed an elaborate membership structure for the steering committee. The plan is to have one Community of Practice, linking all the cohorts. Each cohort elects four members the year they finish the programme, which drops to two members the second year after graduation, as new cohorts graduate and move into the community and onto the committee. Eventually, an advisory committee might be created as well.

Cava has already acted, in a small way, in an EXTRA Community of Practice; she and two other Toronto-based fellows organised a daylong session to introduce the concept of evidence-informed decisions to about 120 managers in their three organisations, an event that was more effective for being collective, she thinks. But she wonders about whether the larger Community of Practice will work. 'I think we will link individually around issues and topics in our regions. If I need something I will pick up the phone', she says, adding 'the Community of Practice wasn't our idea, it was part of the curriculum, something the Foundation wanted to do to make sure connections would live on'. She thinks that could affect its success. 'It didn't germinate with us, there wasn't a groundswell movement. If it's something you really want and really need, you will do it, but when someone else says you should have this, it's a bit artificial'.

Probably the greatest challenge for a national Community of Practice is Canada's two official languages. Foundation-sponsored events all have simultaneous translation, but it is expensive and impractical in most day-to-day life. Certainly, translating everything fellows might want to share, from web postings and journal articles to podcasts and conference calls, is impossible. Francophones are more likely to be bilingual than anglophones, but many of the French-speaking fellows have limited English. Carl Taillon, assistant director general of medical and university affairs at the Centre hospitalier universitaire de Québec, whose English is very good, says it is just easier to talk to another francophone. He thinks working on common topics is what will make a Community of Practice happen. Because he looked at safety in his intervention project, he sees himself connecting with fellows also interested in it, rather than the full group.

Gaetan Tardif, a Montreal-born doctor who is vice president of patient care and chief medical officer at the Toronto Rehabilitation Centre, says culture is more likely than language to keep Quebec fellows from participating in a Community of Practice. Quebec professional organisations offer excellent support to their members, and people in the province do not habitually turn to the rest of Canada for information. Language is no barrier for Tardif, but when he moved to Ontario, Quebec organisations dropped him from their mailing lists, although he was still paying dues and he feels as excluded from Quebec's world of health care as any anglophone. 'You would expect this crew would maybe transcend that a little bit and rise above it, but you also have to contend with busy lives and established patterns and habits', he says.

Next steps

Does all this mean an EXTRA Community of Practice is doomed to failure? Not necessarily. Wenger says that CHSRF's planned annual events, dedicated staff and technological support could be what it takes to sustain a thriving Community of Practice. 'If the Foundation is serious about building a cadre of people who are going to be change agents as a national network, and is willing to put the resources in, it might work (Wenger)', he says.

Meanwhile, the steering committee is exploring several ideas to make the Community of Practice dynamic and useful for its members. One is to use the desktop to explore themes the fellows are interested in, possibly using the Foundation's 2007 campaign on quality in Canadian health care as a pilot project to test ways of linking fellows quickly to new research in their fields. Interactive webcasts, showcasing evidence and featuring an expert, or panel of experts and allowing fellows to ask questions, are other suggestions for keeping fellows linked. The committee will also look into partnerships with health organisations that are already using the web's distance-learning features effectively, which would link EXTRA fellows into existing Canadian health knowledge networks.

But the steering committee does not want those broader links to be just electronic. Because of the mix of partners behind EXTRA, and the fellow's professional affiliations, there are already natural bonds to many health groups in Canada; the steering committee is also exploring ways to get EXTRA fellows and their intervention projects featured at more national events. That will increase opportunities for the face-to-face meetings fellows want, help fellows pursue their diverse interests and begin to integrate the Community of Practice into the larger health care community in Canada.

Because linking to the broader community is the final, essential step in the cultural transformation needed before finding, assessing and using evidence is an essential part of every health care decision. The Canadian Health Services Research Foundation and its partners in EXTRA are committed to the idea that giving health care managers the knowledge, experience and skills to use research effectively will let them improve health services and build a better health care system for Canada. And the partners understand that means the work of promoting research use must go beyond the organisations where EXTRA fellows work. EXTRA, despite its national reach, long-term funding, excellent faculty, high-quality programme and fellows who are the stars of their organisations, can reach only 25 or so new fellows a year. It is through a vibrant and effective Community of Practice, whose members know, firsthand, that training in evidence-based decision making should be standard for leaders in health care, so they can imbue it in the culture of their organisations and the practice of those who work in them that the real transformation of Canada's health system can take place.

Chapter 3

THE INTERIOR HEALTH NURSE PRACTITIONER COMMUNITY OF PRACTICE: FACILITATING NP INTEGRATION IN A REGIONAL HEALTH AUTHORITY

Linda Sawchenko

How it all began

In August 2005, following a number of years of planning, the British Columbia (BC) government passed legislation allowing the introduction of Nurse Practitioners (NPs) into the health care system. Recognising the challenges and struggles that the NP role had faced across Canada, the introduction of this new role into Interior Health communities was intentionally managed through the Professional Practice Office with dedicated leadership and resources provided for the project. Planning for the introduction of this important new role took over a year and involved an initial extensive review of both national and international literature in order to identify the barriers and facilitators to successful integration of the NP role.

Stars aligned

Around the same time as BC government legislated for the introduction of NPs into practice, a new 2-year fellowship programme (Executive Training for Research Application – EXTRA) was launched by the Canadian Health Services Research Foundation to optimise the use of research evidence in managing Canadian health organisations. I was accepted onto the programme for senior nurse, physician and health service executives and used it as an opportunity to focus more on my work on the development of an evidence-informed approach to the introduction of the NPs within Interior Health. As often happens in life, all of this coincided with yet another initiative – this one though was focused specifically on NPs (the Canadian Nurse Practitioner Initiative (CNPI) funded by the Health Canada Primary Health Care Transition Fund) and provided an excellent source of up-to-date research evidence to underpin my project.

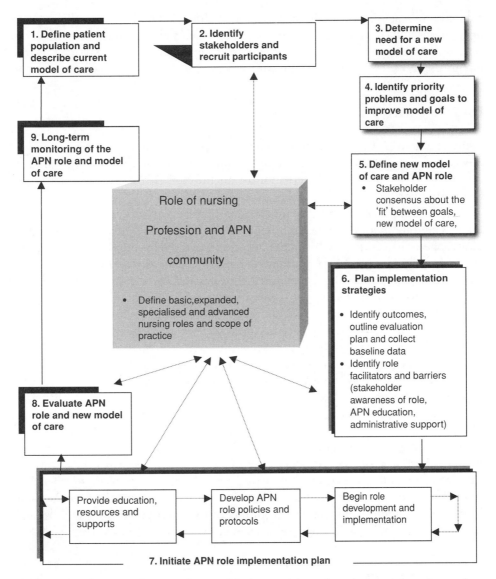

Figure 3.1 The PEPPA framework: a participatory, evidence-based, process for advanced practice nursing (APN) role development, implementation and evaluation. Reproduced from Bryant-Lukosius & DiCenso, copyright 2004 with permission of Blackwell Publishing Ltd.

Based on this extensive review of the literature, it was clear that a consistent approach to the introduction of NPs was critical. To support communities interested in recruiting an NP, the participatory, evidence-based, patient-focused process for advanced practice nursing role development, implementation and evaluation (PEPPA) framework (Bryant-Lukosius & DiCenso, 2004) (Figure 3.1) was used by programme directors to assess their patient populations and identify gaps in the current model of care in order to decide if they really needed an NP and to identify barriers and facilitators to the integration of the NP. Funding was allocated to programmes where these critical early steps had clearly been addressed and where there was evidence of readiness on the part of key stakeholders to work towards integrating NPs into primary health care services.

Evidence into practice

Using Hamric's (2005) work, Interior Health recognised that the new NPs would be novice practitioners and would therefore require support in practice if the initiative was to work – this led to the creation of an Interior Health Nurse Practitioner Community of Practice.

Facilitating the development of an ongoing support network, the 'Nurse Practitioner Community of Practice' and planning for professional development opportunities became a critical factor in the implementation plan. Etienne Wenger in the 2006 class of the EXTRA programme defined *Communities of Practice* (CoP) as 'Groups of people who share a concern or a passion for something they do and learn how to do it better as they interact regularly. They build relationships as they pursue their interests that enable them to learn from each other'. According to Wenger, CoP are formed by people who engage in a process of collective learning in a shared domain of human endeavour: a tribe learning to survive, a band of artists seeking new forms of expression, a group of engineers working on similar problems, a clique of pupils defining their identity in the school, a network of surgeons exploring novel techniques. In this project it was a group of NPs sharing successes and challenges as they pioneered their new role in BC health care system.

The challenge of integrating CoP in an organisation was described by Wenger as an exercise in paradox. How does the organisation engage with them without attempting to control them? In the case of Interior Health, it seems that rather than control the CoP they provided an innovative space within which the NPs could develop their identity and so move from novice to expert practitioners whilst also integrating into primary health care services in BC.

Early, small wins

It is now over 2 years since this CoP started and there are significant signs of early success. Although the number of NPs hired remains small, the effect these individuals are beginning to have in practice is huge. The following stories from Interior Health NPs begin to capture that impact:

> A male patient walked into the health center complaining of neck pain, he was 5 days post biking accident … his request was to 'get something for neck strain pain'. On examination a number of symptoms were found that were not consistent with a neck strain. I explained to the patient that he needed to go to

emergency for evaluation...he refused to go. I shared a story with him about a patient who awoke 7–10 days post injury and was a paraplegic. He finally agreed to go to emergency but still refused the ambulance. I called his friend who agreed to drive him to emergency. The emergency physician called later in the day and said the patient had a fracture dislocation of C5, 6 and 7 which was unstable...they immediately applied tongs and traction and he was sent to a neurosurgeon for bone grafting and application of rods. The patient later returned to me saying that my taking the time to convince him to go to emergency saved him from a wheelchair and may have saved his life.

I was seeing a patient who had developed multiple health concerns over a period of several years and was very depressed about the state of her health. She felt that she had 'tried everything' and so did her physician. After seeing her several times I proposed a referral to a specialist. After going to that appointment, the patient came back to see me and told me that she had new hope to go on. She indicated to the specialist that seeing the NP in her clinic had 'saved her life' because she would never have been willing to try another approach to the way her care was managed without the time taken by the NP to discuss her health plan with her. The consultant's letter returned to the clinic with a note outlining the specialist's acknowledgement of the role the NP had played in delivering care to the patient.

Working as a nurse practitioner, I have had an opportunity to meet many wonderful patients and families. One particular family, struggling with several personal health and economic challenges comes to mind. In the time I have known this family; they have managed to overcome many obstacles. The patient's source of income had run out and she could not work due to chronic pain issues. She was suffering from multiple chronic health problems, each compounding the other. In addition to her health challenges, she was stressed about finances and an inability to contribute to the household income and this caused her to feel depressed. I worked with this patient to identify her personal priorities and to set personal goals. She now has the tools to better manage her pain and has returned to work. She has transportation options available and therefore does not feel isolated and dependent on others. She has begun to exercise and has lost over 10 pounds in one month. Because of this weight loss, which she has struggled with for many years, she is closer to her target weight for knee replacement surgery. She states she now has hope – there is 'a light at the end of the tunnel'. And more importantly, she feels that she does not have to navigate through the health care system on her own – she has an advocate and co-pilot. As a nurse practitioner, I have the opportunity to provide collaborative care to patients and families.

Physicians who work with the NPs are so impressed with their excellent leadership and team-working skills and their willingness to ask questions and learn in order to improve their knowledge and skill base that they 'can't imagine why other physicians wouldn't refer to an NP'. One family physician stated that he has never been happier in his career than he was now having an NP to collaborate with. He is convinced that his patients were receiving better care through this new model of primary health care service. When asked how he would quantify that 'better care', he responded that it is 'easy to see, the patients are no longer in hospital as often or as long'. The British Columbia Ministry of Health has also just recognised the success of our NP programme in improving NP/physician collaborative practice by presenting us with the 'Innovations in Health Care Best Practices' award.

Key to our early successes has been the power of the NP CoP within Interior Health. This CoP has provided significant support to each of the NPs who are generally working as novice practitioners in a new role and as the lone NP in a community. Having the opportunity to share challenges as well as successes has allowed the NPs to learn with and from each other and connect around issues common to the role regardless of setting. The work of the group has included development of communication tools related to the NP role, work on continuing education tools and support to each other in preparing for registration examinations. The community is also providing a support network to this year's new NP graduates who will be beginning their NP practice in Interior Health.

Voices of the NPs in the CoP

Participants were invited to join the CoP and stated that they were immediately 'excited to be able to meet together as a group on a regular basis' because 'the idea of a Community of Practice made sense, both personally and to support others that were developing similar programmes in their areas'. Recently, I conducted a short survey to assess the effectiveness of the CoP, and as you can see from the results in Boxes 3.1 and 3.2, the Interior Health NP Community of Practice has provided not only support for the seven NPs involved but it has also enabled them to develop

---

Box 3.1   The individual benefits of being part of the Community of Practice

'Wonderful opportunities to learn from one another's experience and expertise'
'A sense of "belonging", support and understanding as I work through the growing pains and challenges of blazing the trail for a new profession in B.C.'
'Personal growth'
'Support both professionally and collegially, information, clinical updates'
'Support, Collegiality, Knowledge sharing, Partnership, Friendships'
'Meeting other NPs in IH and having an idea as to who to contact for further info . . . networking'

Box 3.2 The difference that being in the Community of Practice has made

'Being a part of the Community of Practice has provided me with a safe and secure place to share my experiences of being a new NP, and a wonderful opportunity to learn from my peers. These "learnings" have included clinical practice skills, integrating my role into the community, new and innovative programmes and approaches to care'.

'It has made a huge difference. In 19 years of practice, many of them being in advanced practice, I have never been involved in a group that has achieved so many "small wins". This has set the foundation for success not just with my own programmes, but programmes throughout Interior Health. The real benefit has improved patient care throughout the region'.

'It is very important because it decreases the isolation which comes with a new position and a new role'.

'Being involved in our CoP has assisted me in my new role transition and integration. Although I have worked as an NP in the past, the CoP has assisted me in sharing concerns, barriers, issues, and knowledge bringing forth our individual strengths and welcoming new roles/NPs. At times one can feel "on their own" or alone in this new role to BC, the CoP assists in creating a feeling of "belonging"'.

---

their identity through establishing and sharing good practice and stories of success as well as challenges.

Participants in the CoP could easily identify aspects of the CoP that had worked. These ranged from having a facilitator/leader to sharing the work out among the group. They highlighted the usefulness of frequent communications via e-mail and quarterly face-to-face meetings each of which had agenda items agreed beforehand. At the meetings the NPs discussed issues that they were facing – having other NPs, rather than colleagues from other specialisms or disciplines to talk to, was extremely helpful. This helped to create 'the cohesiveness of the entire group with the ultimate goal of improving outcomes for our patients and families. We have all worked on projects both individually and collectively to meet this goal'.

In addition to creating a 'real sense of community', this cohesiveness resulted in some major accomplishments for the CoP which included hosting the first NP conference in BC setting the standard for NPs in the province and inspiring many others (see Box 3.3 for evidence of this) as it brought together almost all of the practicing NPs in the province for a day of sharing, learning and celebration.

Having the CoP might have also been instrumental in attracting new NPs to the region because it was seen as a mechanism for successfully integrating NPs into practice in Interior Health and providing NPs with contacts and networking opportunities as well as those more focused on learning.

Box 3.3 Comments from conference participants

'I found this conference to be the highlight since my graduation as an NP in November 2006. I cannot express how helpful it was to connect with colleagues and to learn of the exciting possibilities ahead for this role. It helped me not feel as isolated as a new practitioner'.
'I am not alone! Inspirational'.
'Inspirational and sense of "community" of NP's – the networking'.
'I hope that as this group grows more, more of the NP's will present and share their work'.
'Inspirational opportunity to meet the other BC NP pioneers'.
'This was an excellent forum for sharing/learning about NP practices in BC'.
'I learned how to start planning and setting groundwork for new NP roles in my community'.
'I will try and stimulate this inspiration and excitement in our HA'.
'Next year it would be good to hear about a role that was not supported and then what was put in place to change that'.

One CoP participant highlighted a major triumph of the CoP as 'our uniqueness in the fact that we are such a close knit sharing group'. But in addition to this, the CoP did share its knowledge with others through a bimonthly clinical update for NPs and also encouraged NP students to participate in order to help them learn the NP role.

Participants were more reluctant to highlight aspects of the CoP that had not worked often stating that they could not think of any. However, when pressed they highlighted the impracticalities for them of having 'shared chairperson responsibilities – because all participants are very busy with a heavy work load and role development in their respective positions' preferring the responsibility to rest on one person's shoulders for a given period of time. They also suggested that perhaps a more formal list of 'action items', with the individual responsible for the action clearly indicated might result in more effective functioning and also provide an opportunity for timelier follow-up of issues. In order to improve the effectiveness of the CoP, they wanted to continue to work on improving access to clients and other smaller goals that could be achieved quickly, whilst still contributing to the larger goal of improved patient care.

Clearly, this CoP has a future. When asked how they saw the CoP developing the participants, almost all saw it growing over time as they welcomed new NPs to Interior Health and to the CoP. Some saw the CoP, whilst keeping its focus on 'setting and achieving goals and integrating ourselves into the current health care system', branching out and becoming involved in research and publication which in turn would aid 'in the success of the NP's new role!' And others continued to see it as a central mechanism for connecting and supporting NP students and themselves.

Perhaps the success of the CoP is best summed up in the words of one of its members:

> It has been a pleasure to be a part of the CoP. I am privileged to be a part of such a dynamic, supportive group. I know this has been demonstrated to other health authorities from our NP conference and the word is out. The CoP is definitely a drawing card for new NPs as one can see the closeness and support we are offered here in Interior Health.

Conclusions and next steps

The current level of success in the Interior Health Nurse Practitioner implementation programme may not have been seen without the preliminary work done, reviewing the literature and the establishment of an implementation plan based on those published research findings. The facilitation of a very effective NP CoP has been critical to the successes we are experiencing with the integration of NPs into working communities around the health authority. The CoP has allowed us, as Thomas Fulton, Professional Practice Leader and Chief of Nursing at Interior Health says, to make 'the consistent connection between practice, operations and evidence . . . the pillars of success behind the Interior Health Nurse Practitioner Integration'.

Chapter 4

DEVELOPING DERMATOLOGY OUTPATIENT SERVICES THROUGH A COMMUNITY OF PRACTICE

Judith Lathlean and Michelle Myall

The idea of a dermatology Community of Practice

Communities of Practice (CoPs) have been promoted as vehicles for bringing together the relevant stakeholders to achieve an agreed task whilst drawing on a range of resources and sources of knowledge. They represent one approach for inter-agency working in which several agencies can be involved in different types of care and can collaborate in both service design and delivery (Lathlean & le May, 2002). This chapter focuses on the successes and challenges of developing, piloting and evaluating a CoP that was established to improve dermatology outpatient services, an initiative that ran alongside another CoP – for developing ear, nose and throat (ENT) outpatient services (see Chapter 8). Both CoPs were facilitated and evaluated by a university-based project team comprising two facilitators and two evaluators/researchers.

The idea for a CoP for dermatology, with an overall aim of taking forward services external to institutional care, was first explored in a 'Consensus Conference' in February 2001 involving a range of participants – policy-makers, managers, clinicians, practitioners and service user organisations – all of whom had a role in dermatology outpatient services. The conference provided an opportunity for both deliverers and consumers of outpatient services to brainstorm and articulate areas of concern and served to clarify the part that a multi-professional group could play in service development in this specific arena. The attendees prioritised 'changing roles within specialised outpatient services' as an important area for a CoP to be constructed around.

Running and evaluating the CoP

A series of four 1-day workshops from June to December 2001 was planned, to be held at the Kings Fund Centre in central London, since this was felt to be a location which could be accessed relatively easily by most potential members. The venue was also chosen because there were good facilities including a library and information resources on site.

The dermatology CoP was to be facilitated by a member of the project team with a view to promoting an environment in which shared learning, partnership and collaboration between the facilitators and CoP participants could take place. The role of the facilitator was to enable the CoP to develop a framework for shared decision making and action between consumers, designers and providers of health care and determine ways in which the outcomes from the CoP working could be transferred from the CoP to the realities of practice (Lathlean & le May, 2002).

In addition, the CoP workshops were to be observed by an evaluator who recorded the development and workings of each meeting and carried out interviews with participants in-between each CoP. As members were likely to be geographically dispersed, it was decided that interviews would be conducted by telephone. At each interview, they were asked to describe the previous meeting, their role within the group and the role of other members. They were also invited to share any views about the pros and cons of the CoP from their perspectives and their expectations of the next meeting. As the project sought to consider the use of knowledge within and by the CoP in relation to its explicit goal, observations of meetings and interviews with participants also explored issues such as knowledge brought to the group, how that knowledge was incorporated into the task and the types of knowledge valued and rejected by participants.

In terms of membership, clearly clinicians would be at the core of the CoP and these could include consultant dermatologists, specialist registrars, clinical assistants, nurses with a specialist interest, practitioners working in primary care (such as the general practitioner – GP). Furthermore, it was important to include managers of dermatology outpatient services and, in line with the imperative to involve service users or consumers more overtly in service development, their engagement in the CoP was also vital. Although it was hoped that the CoP would achieve work of relevance to the UK, for pragmatic reasons, the initial members were to be targeted from within one region of the country.

The series of workshops

Invitations were sent out to encourage attendance at the inaugural workshop for the Outpatient Improvement Communities of Practice. Participants for the dermatology CoP composed two consultant dermatologists, a clinical nurse manager and assistant service manager for dermatology. Whilst some members had attended the consensus conference and decided to continue their participation, others had been nominated by a colleague who had been present at the consensus conference.

The proceedings began with the facilitator explaining to all of the participants the origins of the idea of Communities of Practice to support and develop outpatient services, the structure and purpose of the CoPs and the roles of the facilitator and evaluator. The deliberations of the consensus conferences were discussed highlighting the general topics for possible development that had been forthcoming. Importantly, though, the facilitator tried to convey the purpose of this first workshop as encouraging group members to take ownership of the concept, to construct themselves as a CoP and, as the initial stage of this process, to identify a priority task that they wished to focus on and for which they considered that the group could utilise their knowledge, skills and experience.

There then followed a brainstorming session to identify key issues for outpatient services. Two themes appeared to emerge strongly from this discussion: multidisciplinary training to facilitate role change and the management of outpatient waiting lists and, at the conclusion of the day, the group decided that the development of training, which is multidisciplinary and can address new roles, would be a suitable focus for future meetings. In order to work on this topic, the group decided that other people needed to be recruited to the CoP, including a GP, a specialist nurse, other medical colleagues and a link with a specific medical school, as well as someone who could focus on the patient perspective. Other ideas of participants, such as a pharmacist and a surgeon, were floated as possibilities for later. The participants agreed who would approach these additional people.

The dermatology CoP met on three more occasions within workshops during that year. In July, the second workshop was held and attended by three members from the inaugural meeting, as well as two new participants: a clinical dermatologist and a dermatology nurse specialist. As a result of knowledge brought by the new members, it was decided to refine the original task and revise the focus to identifying and mapping the current position in relation to training and development within dermatology outpatient services, identifying the needs and gaps in provision and to make recommendations which could inform national standards. Furthermore, members agreed that whilst their work needed to concentrate on the region, since this was a regionally orientated group and the knowledge needed to be of local use and application, it was important that the outcomes could be transferred beyond the region and have national relevance. With the task fixed, the remainder of the second session was spent identifying existing resources and the sources of knowledge that needed to be tapped to carry the work forward.

The third and fourth CoP workshops were held in October and December, respectively. The membership on each occasion varied, but there was a core group entailing a consultant dermatologist, a GP, a specialist nurse and a patient representative who attended most meetings. During the workshops they worked on materials gathered between meetings and brought to the session by the participants, and gradually moved towards a decision to develop a 'package' of resources related to the training of staff within a dermatology outpatient setting.

The third meeting was particularly important, not only in terms of further refinement of the task, identifying additional resources and agreeing on its outcomes, but also because probably for the first time members began to see the value and potential impact of the work they were undertaking within the CoP. For example, it was felt that as there was no one source of information which covered the resources available for training and current models and innovations, a 'map' of this would be helpful for both local and national planning and policy-making.

By the fourth workshop, it was evident that the participants were beginning to take ownership of the task. The meeting was spent reviewing the resources that had been identified and brought to the group, as well as finalising outcomes for the project. Members agreed that the resources they had collated should be posted on a website including, for example, publications, reports from working groups, contact points, curricula and existing training resources. Possible hosts for the website were discussed. The group was also keen that the NHS Region Research and Development Directorate, who had funded the project, should take some ownership as well, and it was agreed that regional representatives would be invited to attend a final meeting to launch the resource pack. Members' concerns that constraints on their time would result in an incomplete set of resources at the launch were appeased by the facilitator who suggested employing a researcher to undertake some of the outstanding work. By the end of the meeting, participants had decided upon a date, venue and list of people to be invited to the launch and agreed to attend a further meeting prior to the launch at which they would brief the researcher and confirm the programme for the launch.

The reality of the dermatology CoP

The account of proceedings so far may sound straightforward and the outcomes are largely positive. However, the reality was far from so.

What is a CoP?

One of the first problems for the facilitator was how to convey to a group of clinicians and managers the essence and purpose of, and the expected outcomes from, their engagement in a CoP. These were busy people, often driven by targets but also by a desire to provide the best possible service for clients with limited resources. From the outset it was evident that some struggled with the concept of the CoP. There was a high degree of resistance to the idea of the CoP, and several were confused about what it was and how it would 'work' effectively. The facilitator, especially in the first workshop, was faced with strong opposition from some participants who repeatedly sought to put obstacles in the way and generally make life difficult. In an attempt to appease the concerns of the CoP group, the facilitator shared their own dislike for the term 'Community for Practice' and suggested that they could decide if they continued to call themselves a 'Community of Practice' or eventually lost the name.

The lack of clarity, and in some cases scepticism about what could be achieved, was also expressed in the initial interviews of participants. It was evident that despite one of the hopes of the participants for the inaugural meeting being 'to understand 'CoP' jargon', there continued to be strong objections for the term by some members who dismissed it as a phrase they 'disliked immensely'. For example, one participant described the name 'Community of Practice' as 'meaningless [because it] makes little immediate sense to most people' and they had little hesitation in admitting that they considered it to be 'one of the most horrid terms [they'd] come across in [their] experience in medical management'. This participant's dislike of the term 'CoP' was reinforced by their avoidance of using it, instead employing the strategy whereby they continually asked the interviewer to repeat it, which prevented them from having to articulate the phrase. In addition, some members continued to be somewhat cynical regarding the potential of the CoP to achieve something meaningful:

> It remains to be seen whether people are going to participate or not, so I still have some scepticism and I suspect others may have as well. I'm not entirely sure whether the agenda of the people who set up the project matches the agenda of the people who're participating in the project so that'll be interesting. [Dermatology Consultant]

In effect, very quickly the participants tended to refer to themselves as the 'dermatology' group, rather than a CoP, so as they proceeded, it was not a major issue.

What do facilitators and evaluators do?

Another issue was the respective roles of the facilitator and evaluator and their relationship to the group. For example, the facilitators for the CoP were seen as being part of a research project, working with their own agenda, and several members appeared to think that the evaluator was present simply to minute the meetings and made reference to this right up until the final workshop. This view of facilitators as 'leading the show' was difficult to shift. Participants in the dermatology CoP appeared to veer between wanting them to lead, to feeling resentful that they as recipients were 'guinea pigs' in a kind of social-engineering experiment. Thus, for the facilitators, getting the balance right and trying to encourage members to see that what they considered to be important and achievable should be the prime focus proved to be very challenging.

Furthermore, the absence of a preset topic by the facilitator and the realisation that they as participants would be required to identify a task relating to an area they considered to be important for dermatology was a difficult concept for most members to take on board. As the following quotation suggests, some members struggled with the idea that they had been brought together for what they deemed 'no specific purpose' and not in response to a 'perceived need':

> I come from a school which says you don't set something up and then see what it can do; you identify an objective and then you decide what you need in order to achieve that objective. Now we've done that exactly the wrong way round because we've set up the community of practice thing and said 'now what can we do with it?' and so we're desperately looking for an objective. [Service User Representative]

How important is structure?

As the workshops progressed, it was evident that participants responded well to having an agenda and structure for meetings because this was the manner in which they were used to working. CoP members perceived structure in a positive way and worked more productively within defined parameters. Consequently, they were uncomfortable with any lack of structure, and without it the meetings were seen to lack purpose. When structure was present decisions were made, and when it was absent this often led to a lack of focus, frustration and a questioning of the aims and motives of the research project. The need for structure was reflected in participants' interviews. For example:

> I think [each meeting needs an agenda], a reminder of what people said they were going to do, it focuses people, stops people going off on different tangents or re-doing things again … I would want to get some more structure now into the meetings, you know who is coming, who isn't coming, identify the gaps of our knowledge or skills – gaps that we're missing, give enough notice of meetings for the future, clarify the task, who's going to be doing what, find a chairman, find some finishers, so those are the sorts of things that one would do if we were going to take it further. [Dermatology Consultant]

The ideal size and membership of the group

The size of the CoP was commented upon by members initially with a 'disappointment that there were so few people' and an expectation of a larger group. This was viewed as potentially hindering the work of the CoP in terms of skill mix and level of influence to take things forward:

> Well I think the problem was that you didn't have enough people to start with so I still don't think there's the groundwork to pull together a group of people who could work [or] would be able to take something forward. [Dermatology Consultant]

> There's always that fear that a small group of people are just a blip on the horizon and actually we could put a lot of effort and work into this but we're [just] reinventing the wheel or at the end of the day too small to take anything forward, we're just too small a group to have an influence. [Outpatient Service Manager]

However, by the third meeting of the CoP the size of the group was perceived as an advantage and by the fourth some suggested that it was the combination of size and composition of the group that was important. Also, it was felt that a small group was preferable as it avoided role duplication:

> Well I like small groups; any more than six and I think the returns on it are in inverse proportions. I found it was actually a very good group because there were … four or five of us … who all came from different perspectives. [GP]

> I think it's also easier when you have smaller numbers and when you have participants from their different disciplines rather than duplicating that. I think that when you get duplication then each group has to negotiate its position, what it's interested in, who's going to lead, what roles everyone's going to play. [Dermatology Consultant]

As a result of participants' recognition for the need of additional knowledge and expertise, new members were invited to join the CoP. The implications of changing membership were felt to alter the team dynamics. For example, the introduction of someone in the same role type as an existing member appeared to affect the latter's contribution. The nurse member from the first CoP meeting became more vocal and participated to a greater extent in the second CoP in which another dermatology nurse was present, and she said, 'I did appreciate [name of nurse] being there because it was like a support mechanism'. The shifting of allegiances between existing members was also noted to the extent that when certain people were present, an existing member tended to 'bow' to the new member's point of view, possibly because they were seen to be more powerful or more knowledgeable.

Participants sometimes appeared irritated that new members needed to be brought up to speed and that they 'had to go back over old ground' which they felt could hinder the progress of the CoP:

> I think the difficulty is when you have new people in a group and then you have other existing people who have already been there, it's trying to make sure everybody's caught up to the same point and so that those who are new you've got to bring into the group and those who are already there, you've got to keep, and it's a challenge. [Outpatient Services Manager]

Although the continuity of the group could be fractured by its changing composition; nevertheless, the group recognised that bringing new people is also meant the introduction of new ideas, an important aspect of a CoP striving to promote new knowledge. However, this process needed 'managing':

> It affects the continuity but everybody new coming in naturally comes up with new ideas and while I'm not disputing that you need new ideas . . . what happens to the old ones, you can't take them all on board, you have to be quite strict with what you're going to achieve and what you're going to look at and how. So I think it's difficult with the group members changing and introducing new people. [Dermatology Nurse Specialist]

How did the CoP's members learn from each other?

Within the CoP different sources and types of knowledge were used by members when working on the tasks. The sources of information included other medical colleagues, university curricula for professionals specialising in dermatology, parliamentary and other reports relating to dermatology and research papers. The types of knowledge were varied and heavily reliant on personal and experiential knowledge exposed in storytelling, factual medical and clinical knowledge, empirical knowledge derived from research sources and managerial knowledge gained from their roles as managers. Knowledge brought to the group was shared within the CoP through a variety of means which included individual members volunteering narratives of personal and professional experiences, often illustrated with examples, specific members being asked by the facilitator or other CoP participants for information they were believed to hold and members introducing different types of knowledge that were then expanded or build upon by other CoP members. Often knowledge was shared verbally rather than visually by participants, and whilst this worked well for some, others felt that it was not the most productive way for the group to transfer knowledge:

> I came away from that meeting in June feeling that there was going to be information shared that would be of value in the future but I think even before that last meeting if I'd sat down and put my head round it then it was a case of thinking we needed to be looking at something visually, using the board, rather than [just] talking. [Outpatient Services Manager]

It was evident that knowledge acquired from inside the CoP sometimes was shared outside, for example, at health care trust meetings or less formally in conversations with colleagues. Furthermore, as participants developed greater enthusiasm for the project and took it on board, they began to recognise that the knowledge gained within the CoP could be used outside of the group to improve dermatology services and inform others of the existing resources for dermatology training. As one member suggested:

> It's important to have something to put into practice, something we can all take back to our areas and put into [use]. [Clinical Nurse Manager]

During the workshops sources of knowledge were often ignored or under-utilised by the CoP members. This included information brought to the meetings by existing members as part of their 'homework' tasks, as well as knowledge introduced by new members. Whilst some participants considered that the non-utilisation of such sources to be 'par for the course', others felt that it was a waste:

> I was thinking that the documentation that the nurse and one of the consultants brought to the meeting was referred to but wasn't really touched on which I think was difficult because they had obviously put a lot of work into what they produced . . . [New members] also brought a lot of knowledge and experience and contact but I think we did not sufficiently plan beforehand how we could use their knowledge. [Outpatient Services Manager]

The rejecting or neglecting of particular knowledge sources was to some extent linked to the CoP members valuing and trusting certain types above others. On the whole, the knowledge that they tended to be most confident about was derived from people and bodies they saw as 'experts', such as clinicians and professional organisations like the British Association of Dermatologists, as well as those which were, in their view, 'evidence-based'. Conversely, there was an overwhelming distrust of information provided on internet websites and through the media and by 'complementary practitioners' who were considered not 'to have much to offer medicine' because of the lack of an evidence base. Scepticism towards such sources of knowledge also militated against inviting certain types of representatives to join the CoP. For example, there was opposition towards both patients and 'complementary therapists' becoming part of the group, and it was agreed that the CoP should 'confine itself to the professional'. This was an interesting conclusion for the group to reach in relation to patients, given that an original intention had been to gain the 'user' or 'consumer' view within the CoP and therefore to include representatives of consumers.

The outcomes of the CoP

With the help of the researcher, who was employed for a set period of time to assist with collating resources and information relating to the training and development of dermatology health care professionals, the CoP participants produced a resource pack which comprised a series of electronic documents, summaries, abstracts and other information relevant to training and development, cross-referenced to the original sources. In order to ensure the resource pack was accessible at both a local and national level, members agreed that it should be made available on websites hosted by one or more dermatology organisations.

The launch for the resource pack was held in March 2002 at the King's Fund Centre, London, and was attended by representatives from the Department of Health, dermatology organisations such as the British Association of Dermatologists and NHS trust personnel nationally. The programme for the event included an overview of the dermatology Community of Practice presented by the facilitator, followed by a session on the context for the group's work led by the core CoP members. Then there was a presentation about the process of developing the electronic resource pack and a demonstration of it in action by the researcher. The launch ended with an open discussion where all participants were encouraged to consider the part they could play in developing an action plan for setting up, accessing and managing the website on which the electronic resources would be placed.

Whilst the electronic resource pack represented a significant and worthwhile outcome from the dermatology CoP, it was evident that there were other, less tangible ones as well. By the time of the launch, the CoP members had taken ownership of the task and recognised that they had produced a product that was innovative and could impact positively on their service. This ensured a commitment to taking the resource forward and attempting to secure funding for its ongoing development at both a local and national level. Whilst the members saw no further role for the CoP, and it was generally agreed that the group would dissolve after the launch, they pledged to be part of a stakeholder group responsible for maintaining and updating the website.

In addition, a further outcome was the change in attitudes towards the concept of 'Communities of Practice'. The scepticism and cynicism which had overshadowed the initial workshops were replaced with enthusiasm and a belief in the CoP as an 'excellent model for the NHS'. One member described working in the group as 'an enriching experience' and outlined to the audience at the launch the benefits he had derived from being part of the group, which included the opportunity to network:

It's always interesting to hear the perspective of [other members] and certainly our conversations off camera have been revealing and interesting but for things nothing to do with what we are talking about. It's a sort of networking opportunity and chance to gain information which otherwise one would not acquire. [GP]

Lessons to be learned

Our experience of facilitating and evaluating a dermatology CoP raised a number of key points which could inform similar models of inter-agency working. The lessons to be taken forward are shown in Box 4.1.

In setting up a CoP, it is usually hoped that the efforts and energies of the group will be sustained beyond its formal meetings. In the case of this CoP, the enthusiasm for the working of the group, and the pride regarding the outcomes gained, was palpable. However, even though this was so, perhaps because the members were

---

Box 4.1   Lessons to be taken forward from a constructed inter-agency CoP

- To ensure commitment and continued participation, members need to have a clear understanding of the rationale for bringing them together as a group. Also, they may need reassurance of a shared purpose between the facilitators and themselves.
- It may take time for participants to agree on a task or topic area which they consider to be a worthwhile. The focus may need to be moulded over time for members to see the importance of undertaking work to achieve their goals.
- In the early stages of the CoP, the facilitator may be relied upon to 'lead' the group until a natural leader emerges or is elected by members. In the case of the dermatology, CoP leadership was strongly linked to ownership and it was only when they recognised that they as a group had the power to potentially improve dermatology services that one member put themselves forward for this role.
- The construction of the CoP membership is likely to change during its lifetime as gaps in knowledge and expertise are identified by existing members and new participants are invited to join the group. Whilst changes in membership composition are likely to be important to achieving outcomes, they may also introduce challenges to the group in terms of altering team dynamics and shifting allegiances.
- A CoP may be more likely to succeed in realising its goal if it has a core membership to ensure tasks are completed and who are committed to taking forward the outcome beyond the boundaries of the group.

used to working to an agenda, to finishing 'projects' and then proceeding to the next most urgent task or activity, they looked elsewhere to other avenues for continuation and action. They hoped that an organisation such as the British Association of Dermatologists would take the website on further and there was considerable discussion about this initially. Nevertheless, there was also the need for updating; priorities change in these organisations and resources are limited. Therefore, it could be said that the main enduring successes of the CoP can be thought of as the actual experience of working together and the generation of a tangible CD Rom.

Part 3

GENERATING PROFESSIONAL AND PATIENT CAPITAL

The third part of this book centres on how Communities of Practice (CoPs) contribute (or not) to the generation of professional and patient capital. Chapters 5, 6 and 7 cluster around the theme of professional capital, whilst Chapter 8 concentrates on patient capital.

In Chapter 5, John Gabbay and I draw on the findings from an ethnographic study of doctors working as general practitioners in one English primary care practice. This chapter illustrates how clinicians working in a multidisciplinary CoP develop knowledge and put it into practice and as a consequence build professional capital. Mary Gobbi in Chapter 6 provides some thoughts about how nurses learn in the workplace community and further explores the professional capital theme, using examples from nursing practice to underline the complexity of this way of learning. Whilst Chapter 5 explicitly focused on CoPs and their likely contribution to the development of professional capital, Chapter 6 reminds us that this can happen both within and outwith CoPs and as such is useful in situating CoPs in the development of professional capital. Chapter 7 takes readers on a somewhat different journey. In this chapter, Alex le May considers how CoPs could contribute to the development of health practice in developing countries.

As I have said in the introduction to this book that it is impossible to think about the development of professional capital in health and social care without also considering the development of patient capital. In order to encourage readers to consider how patient capital might be developed in CoP, I have ended this part of the book with a chapter which shows how storytelling was used to generate patient capital in CoPs which brought patients and professionals together to design health and social care services.

Chapter 5

PRACTICE MADE PERFECT: DISCOVERING THE ROLES OF A COMMUNITY OF GENERAL PRACTICE

John Gabbay and Andrée le May

Why, how and where we undertook the study

A lot of time, energy and resources have been expended in the past few decades trying to induce clinicians to make better use of research evidence (e.g. Haines & Donald, 1998; Gray, 2001). The results of these efforts have never lived up to the hopes of those promoting evidence-based practice (e.g. Trinder & Reynolds, 2000). Health services across the world have been frustrated in their attempts to persuade clinicians either to find, appraise and apply the best evidence themselves or to use evidence-based guidelines and treatment protocols. The study described in this chapter began with the premise that this frustration might be because the evidence-based medicine movement has, ironically, paid insufficient attention to the evidence from social science, psychology and philosophy about the nature of knowledge in practice and how it gets used in the real world. In particular, it seemed to us that the idea that one could improve practice simply by somehow delivering better facts to the desks of clinicians who are better trained in the rational use of such facts flew in the face of all the evidence that has accumulated in the past few decades in the literature about organisational knowledge management and CoP (e.g. Nonaka & Takeuchi, 1995; Davenport & Prusak, 1998; Brown & Duguid, 2000). So the aim of our study was to see what actually happens when clinicians put knowledge into practice and whether it perhaps conforms to the more complex social patterns that have been described in such literature. If so, then maybe one could use that insight to inform the continuing attempts to improve the knowledge base of practice.

We therefore undertook an ethnography to identify and describe the individual, social and organisational processes by which primary care clinicians transform the many potential sources of evidence into knowledge in practice. We used ethnography, which is perhaps best described as hanging around with a purpose followed up with intensive analysis of what one has observed (Spradley, 1979; Agar, 1996; Eriksen, 2001), because it seemed to us to be the research method most likely to help understand what really goes on in clinicians' day-to-day practice and how their culture actually works. Readers interested in the detail of methods used in this study should turn to the methodological postscript to this chapter.

We gained access to 'Lawndale', a successful and very highly regarded primary care practice in 'Woodsea', a semi-rural blue-collar town in the south of England with a large elderly population. There are seven partner general practitioners (GPs) – two women and five men whose ages ranged from about 35 to about 60 – plus three salaried sessional GPs and at any one time a GP registrar. Other key clinicians include three practice nurses and a phlebotomist. Between them they have a list of around 12 000 patients of whom 30% are over 65 years old, reflecting the popularity of the area for retirees. Fully computerised in its recently purpose-built premises, Lawndale is exceptionally well organised. The high quality of the practice was confirmed when we learned that three of the partners had recently been awarded prestigious Fellowships by the Royal College of General Practitioners, and when 3 years into our study, the practice also received the College's coveted Quality Practice Award.

During the early part of our ethnography, when we were focusing mainly on the day-to-day clinical work carried out by individual practitioners, we did not appreciate the importance of the informal chats that went on between them, nor of the formal meetings – of which there were plenty. Every month there was a clinical meeting, a staff training meeting, a finance meeting, a treatment room meeting, a receptionists' meeting, an educational meeting (in the form of a lecture open to neighbouring practices too) and a primary health care team meeting. Every week there was an executive meeting of a subset of the partners. In the evenings, monthly there was a partners' meeting (off site, over dinner) and a practice meeting (following a free meal for all attendees who included doctors, nurses and receptionists). Every 2 months were meetings about IT and education; every quarter there was a staff meeting of which one each year was an awayday for all staff. And every month the GPs could also attend an educational evening meeting for all GPs across a much wider area, which gave plenty of scope for networking. There was also a range of committees and other local and national meetings attended by some of the Lawndale partners.

Perhaps we initially missed the significance of all those meetings – not to mention the profusion of informal chats that went on over coffee, in the common room, the treatment room, or on the corridor or other shared spaces, or by popping into each other's offices and surgeries – because we were too engrossed in the individual work of the clinicians. But also we were concerned not to let our prior assumptions about social and organisational knowledge networks and communities affect the rigour of our study of clinical practice by focusing too quickly on these social phenomena. Be that as it may, our initial analysis focused on individual practice – the clinician seeing the patient – and that was where we very quickly made two interesting findings: the range of GPs' roles and the idea of clinical 'mindlines'.

GPs' multiple roles

We soon noticed that clinicians' daily activities slip frequently, effortlessly and unconsciously between many implicit roles. Even in the course of a few minutes, a GP's activities may be informed, e.g. by their role as clinician (e.g. diagnosing, prescribing, advising, explaining, advocating), as manager (e.g. managing resources, personnel and logistics, training staff, developing the IT system, handling the Primary Care Trust, complying with contractual and legal requirements, monitoring and improving quality), by their role in public health (e.g. disease prevention, health promotion, screening), and by what one might call the professional role of developing and maintaining competence (e.g. keeping up to date, reviewing practice, nurturing collegial networks, learning to 'work' the local system, sustaining credibility, representing the interests of one or another group such as one's discipline or practice, teaching and training others). The decision to routinely order a biochemical profile, for example, looks very different through the eyes of a clinician, resource manager, contract monitor, staff trainer, patient advocate, health promoter, and so on. And yet during the course of even one patient consultation, a GP might have to adopt several of these roles. The roles (which are merely examples, neither exhaustive nor mutually exclusive) may overlap; some clinicians play certain roles less than others or even hardly at all; and clinicians vary in how they handle the tensions and potential fragmentation brought about by the conflicting pulls the roles can exert. This multiplicity of roles was to be an important insight that helped explain our subsequent findings.

Clinical mindlines

Watching the clinicians in their day-to-day practice and discussions about work confirmed that in their actual clinical work GPs rely almost exclusively on the knowledge that they already carry in their heads. There is of course nothing surprising in that finding: what else are all those years at medical school, clinical training and continuous professional development designed to do but to inculcate knowledge and patterns of thinking and behaviour that inform the clinicians' practice throughout their professional lives? But this means that clinicians only rarely access, appraise and use explicit evidence directly from research or other formal sources such as guidelines, which in turn means that the relationship between day-to-day practical knowledge and the available sources for updating or amending that knowledge is not direct and linear but indirect and blurred. Any new knowledge that practitioners acquire becomes absorbed into what we have called 'mindlines' – internalised, collectively reinforced, tacit guidelines in the head (Gabbay & le May, 2004). These mindlines are flexible, often working via reasoning akin to 'fuzzy logic' (Zadeh & Yager, 1987) that eschews the hard edges of clinical guidelines and allows for judgement and plasticity in their application. Mindlines are systematically laid down and ingrained during the clinicians' training and are then modified, refined and occasionally completely revised over their professional careers by experience, reading, their interactions with each other and with opinion leaders, patients, pharmaceutical representatives, and other sources of practically oriented and often tacit knowledge. As experience accumulates and organisational roles shift and science advances and guidelines change, so mindlines constantly evolve. More importantly, the complexity of applying any learned routine to varying and often quite complicated individual circumstances means that the art of clinical practice necessarily relies on much more than can ever be fully explained, let alone comprehensively codified in written documents. Thus, the constant crafting and reformulation of clinicians' mindlines is much better suited than written, explicit guidelines could ever be to resolving the highly variable and constantly shifting requirements that shape the way the practitioners, with their multiple roles, can best manage any given disease.

Sources of knowledge

Once we had arrived at that conclusion, the next step was to find out whatever we could about the way individual practitioners' mindlines evolve. It was clear that a great deal depended on clinicians' experience, which moulded and refined their individual mindlines; but what other sources of information helped them to develop their clinical practice, and how? We were keen to ascertain what they read, what sources they referred to (on-line or from books, journals or other written materials), what they felt they learned from continuing professional development or courses, how much was down to experience, and so on. We found it frustrating at first that although the doctors later agreed with our analysis about the way they used 'mindlines' in their day-to-day practice, they found it very difficult to be explicit about the sources of information and evidence that informed and moulded those mindlines. On reflection, however, we concluded that this was not very surprising. After all, one would expect mindlines to be by their very nature complex and multi-layered; as they are built up over many years by accretion and erosion from multiple sources that become almost subliminally absorbed into the clinicians' thinking and practice it would not be surprising that they were hard to untangle. (It would be like asking you the reader to explain in full all the sources of information that have led you to be agreeing or disagreeing with the notion of mindlines . . . .) Nevertheless, we felt it important to try and elicit some more reflections about the sources of information that doctors are expected to use, such as guidelines, research findings, expert systems and protocols.

Those who advocate evidence-based practice expect clinicians to develop their practice in line with the latest reliable scientific research and to behave in a very rational manner. For example, they encourage clinicians faced with a clinical problem to formulate specific questions in order to search the most comprehensive and up-to-date published sources of scientifically verified information, assess how robust and relevant the scientific evidence is, and then apply it judiciously to the patient in whom the question arose. But, although the Lawndale clinicians maintain a high quality of practice, we have never found them following that linear, rational set of actions. Checking some published guidelines when preparing a draft practice policy to be discussed at a meeting is about as close as it ever gets. Despite the plethora of published guidelines available to them in paper form or electronically, we have never once observed the clinicians refer to them during clinical practice – except to point to one of the laminated guidelines on their walls in order to explain something to the patient or to one of us. Nor have we ever seen them try to solve a clinical problem in real time by accessing the expert system available on their computer. Lawndale's sophisticated computer system allows easy direct access to a number of approved expert systems – and more generally to the internet – but it is very rare for the established full-time GPs (unlike, say, trainees) to use them. Their own average estimates at Lawndale are that they might use such facilities less than once every week, and even then it would probably be to download information to give to patients.

They have told us that they do look through guidelines – either in preparation for a practice meeting where they are being expected to bring the practice policy for a given clinical condition up to date, or more informally to ensure that their own practice is generally up to standard. For example, one partner told us that when a new guideline arrived in the post, he would leaf through it – as long as it looked authoritative and well produced – to reassure himself that there was nothing major that needed changing in his practice. If there were, he would discuss it with colleagues before deciding whether to alter what he generally did for patients with that condition.

When necessary, the doctors know where to look for authoritative guidance either on the internet or on published sources, and their choices vary. When, for example, one relatively young partner had to develop a practice protocol for chronic kidney disease, he went on line to consult local and national guidelines and the National Service Framework, did some simple Google searches and looked up reliable web-sites aimed at GPs, some of which were recommended by email discussion groups or magazine articles that colleagues had passed on to him. But when one of the older partners was asked to draft a practice protocol for heart failure, she turned to the local (printed) hospital guidelines produced by a team led by a respected local cardiologist, who, she assumed, had 'drawn upon all the evidence'. (She had recently attended a course run by him on this topic.) These guidelines 'reinforced' her existing practice, but she supplemented them by reading two other sets of published guidelines, just to be sure. She also carried out an audit of Lawndale's current practice, which they knew needed overhauling. All of these were synthesised into the policy she brought to the meeting.

As these examples show, when the doctors do need to check something for a particular purpose such as drafting a policy, they tend to access different sources. But usually, rather than directly accessing new knowledge in the scientific literature, the Lawndale practitioners take shortcuts to keep up to date. As one partner put it, they 'glean' what is thought to be best practice from, e.g., the way local consultants treat their patients, from snippets of reading, and from each other, especially by means of partners with specific areas of expertise helping to keep each other up to date.

They scan many sources, all of which they regard more or less sceptically as being in their different ways potentially unhelpful or misleading. They include the popular doctors' magazines (colloquially called the 'GP comics') mailed free of charge to practices in the UK and skim reading through the many sources of guidance that arrive unsolicited in the mailbox. They also include information put across by representatives of the pharmaceutical industry, but these are treated with considerable scepticism, although that does not necessarily mean they are without influence, as the practitioners themselves admit. To a lesser extent, advice or guidance from the Department of Health and its local representatives is also regarded with suspicion, usually on the grounds that their motives might not be just in the patient's interest but also the NHS budget's. The local pharmaceutical adviser, although he could potentially be tarred with that same brush, has however earned the respect of the practitioners and has been a highly trusted source.

The GPs also meticulously pursue the requirements laid down for continuing professional development (CPD) by, for example, attending courses and lectures and recording in their CPD portfolios what they have gained from so doing. But they find the direct relevance of such activity very variable, and – like the 'gleaning' described above – mainly to be a way of checking whether one's mindline is more or less in line with current thinking. But even that is highly dependent on how well the educational material fits with the GPs' practical concerns. All too often, such educational events are regarded as being rather removed from the realities of practice, the more popular ones being those that keep things simple, relevant and above all practically applicable.

When the information the practitioners have acquired from all these various sources gets discussed, as it frequently does as an integral part of both formal and informal meetings, it is partly to pass it on but partly also to check out each other's views. Practical know-how is an important feature of such chat. Much the most common currency during their many exchanges of information is geared towards telling or showing each other hands-on knowledge, e.g. stories of how they have dealt with clinical problems, demonstrations of how they find and code events on the computer system (and improve data accuracy in so doing), or reviewing their methods for ensuring that patients are dealt with by the right person at the right time. Such discussions on any given topic, especially in the formal practice meetings, tend to slip seamlessly between the GPs' roles – the medical role (e.g. what investigations do), the logistical (who should do them and when), the administrative (how to code it on the computer, how to convey the laboratory results), the reflective role (reviewing the records of patients who have had this procedure), and so on. Clinical guidelines, educational events and other central guidance such as the GP contract documentation, which tend to focus mainly on the clinician's medical role (e.g. what investigations to do), do not fit easily with such a discourse because they usually omit all these other aspects of clinical practice.

Take the example of chronic kidney failure: national guidance, as set out in the new NHS contract with GPs (Department of Health, 2005a, 2006a) suggests that patients with a certain biochemical profile (an estimated glomerular filtration rate, or eGFR, of <60 mL/min/1.73 m^2, in case you were wondering) should be followed up and managed. This requirement sounds perfectly straightforward, but for Lawndale it generated a host of ancillary questions, which were crucial to the decision as to the threshold at which one should diagnose chronic kidney disease. The potentially conflicting roles of general practice were all represented in the ensuing discussion. Would the results of routine screening overburden resources without really improving health? (financial and public health role) Would lots of patients be unnecessarily alarmed? (clinical role) How would it be practicable to carry out all the extra tests? (logistical role) What adverse impact would that have on Lawndale's workload and that of the local specialist services? (managerial role) Such questions, on which practice policy depended, remained unanswered by educational sessions and published guidance. But, being exactly the sorts of questions that mindlines routinely have to encompass alongside the more strictly medical aspects of day-to-day practice, they dominated, and were only answered by, the practitioners' discussions of the topic.

In short, the two main findings from our early ethnography seem to provide two good sets of reasons why GPs are so often dismissive of the research-based guidance they receive from guidelines and other educational materials. Firstly, the GPs already carry the essentials of most such material in their heads in the form of mindlines, which means they are nearly always already familiar with it, or know where to look quickly in order to check and refresh it as needed. And secondly, the received guidance tends to fail to take account of the concerns actually troubling the GP, not least because, unlike mindlines, it underestimates the non-medical roles in a clinician's job. So the clinicians are disinclined to accept such guidance at face value until they check it out with trusted colleagues who understand and share the same practical concerns that require similar mindlines. New information is incorporated into such mindlines not via direct ingestion of the 'expert' views and guidelines – whatever their source – but through discussions and down-to-earth, practical, experientially relevant analyses. And that is where the clinicians' CoP come into the picture.

The Community of Practice

As our ethnography continued, it increasingly seemed to us that ideas were being shared and developed – or as we would put it, mindlines were being checked and refined and hence were evolving – through interactions between colleagues. To really check out what is thought to be the best practice, the GPs tend to turn to the sources that they trust the most, and the most important of these, which provide the most relied-upon and efficient shortcut to the best up-to-date practice, are reached via their professional networks among other doctors. What is the respected local consultant doing with this new anti-diabetic drug? How does the partner who has the lead in diabetes (who can be depended on to do that little bit extra to keep up to date in that specific area) think one should do things these days? What do colleagues think about this new suggestion for treatment, and have they tried it and with what results? It is through these kinds of discussions and interactions with trusted colleagues that any change in practice is most likely to become embedded in their mindlines.

We have observed many examples of mutual consultation between colleagues, each drawing on his or her different sources of knowledge, which demonstrate how important is the level of trust that each clinician is able to put on those sources. Networking is vital in order to know which colleagues and which sources to rely on. A great deal of the social interaction and professional to-ing and fro-ing between doctors/nurses and other practice staff – and beyond – can be seen as a way of checking out who or what are the most authoritative and trustworthy sources (both interpersonal but also written or on-line). But the doctors rarely if ever question how – or even whether – those sources give opinions that are rooted in research evidence. This is simply assumed, because those sources are supposed to be the people in the know. The primary source of such knowledge networks tends to be the immediate group of GPs at the practice, but this is not a simple unitary group. The participants also meet as subgroups either informally or formally, where they may go into more depth over certain topics, and those groups may include others such as the practice nurses and practice manager. (The monthly multidisciplinary practice meetings are where these most broadly and collectively overlap.) The members of these groups have also their own other networks of old colleagues, local clinicians, committees, and so on, who are used as trusted sources of information. In short, there are many loosely overlapping Communities of Practice and related knowledge networks. How, then, do they operate?

Conversations between the GPs around the Lawndale's coffee room are rife with what one partner called 'anecdotes with a purpose'. They chat about experiences with patients, about things they have heard or come across at meetings, in their reading, on the radio, from the pharmaceutical representatives, from patients who have heard about a new treatment, and so on. Each chips in with what they have heard and understood about the topic, or maybe their own experience. One cannot imagine that this could happen without the relaxed gossip, banter and inside jokes that characterise the exchanges. Often amid much humour and mutual de-bunking, they posit their own current practice, telling brief stories about recent patients, occasionally scoring good-natured points over each other, sometimes with admonishments – usually sharp, humorous and elliptical, but sometimes logically explained. Good group dynamics characterised by trust and mutual recognition help them to deal constructively with differing or even conflicting views, to expose problems and deficiencies, agree practical solutions and review them.

This ease of efficient communication is also very evident in the formal practice meetings where protocols have been discussed either – in the early part of our ethnography – in preparation for the Quality Practice Award or more recently to help meet the demands of the new GP contract. At first these meetings were dom-inated by the medical partners and practice manager, but over the years the group dynamics described above have become established among all who attend these meetings, as evidenced not least by the humour at each other's expense, regardless of 'rank'. As a result they have become a very effective forum for doctors, nurses, phlebotomist, receptionists and others, chaired usually by the practice manager, to all engage actively in discussions about the practice. In exchanging and developing ideas on clinical policy, the participants – not least the GPs – are continually exposing and filling gaps in their knowledge, usually by comparing, refining and readjusting not only the way they do clinical work, but also the logistics such as clinic arrangements and computer coding. They often do a 'reality check' against actual case records or against each others' clinical or logistical experience. At such times the discussions in the meetings are swift but sometimes complex. Thus, for example, in 2006 the first discussion on the contractual requirements about chronic kidney disease, with contributions from six of the seven GPs present, took less than 10 minutes, but already foreshadowed, in some detail, almost all of the concerns and conflicts that ran through the later wide ranging debates on this topic, which had important ramifications, as we shall see below.

At such meetings we have been able to see how each participant both contributes knowledge he or she already has about the subject under discussion and also draws from it to amend his or her own mindlines. The participants also bring varied skills and resources to the meeting. Each partner has the lead in a number of clinical fields and will prepare for the meeting by checking up on best practice or contractual requirements (not always considered to be the same thing) and on current Lawndale activity in their designated field as recorded in the computer system. The nurses, phlebotomist and receptionists bring a wealth of knowledge about the locality and individual patients, as well as anecdotes about the variations in GP practices and the administrative consequences. And the participants bring other resources to the meeting. For example, one partner being on a number of local and national committees is also the main source of knowledge about changing NHS requirements and resources; he tends often to have his laptop on with reference material (usually about the GP contract) to hand should it be needed, which is quite rarely. Another will often bring in the local hospital guidelines to help with the discussion and occasionally use them to back up a point she is making. But although explicit reference to written guidance is very rare, as far as anyone can tell all the GPs seem abreast of the main points of current best practice and are somehow generally familiar enough with any guidelines under discussion to criticise them in some detail.

When, for example, the partner who had drafted a protocol for heart failure (as above p. 53) brought it to an early Quality Practice Award meeting, its scientific basis was hardly questioned; rather, it was taken for granted that it was sound and that she had consulted trusted sources (the main one of which, the local hospital guideline, she had indeed brought to the meeting to refer to, if necessary). But they robustly debated the detail, a discussion which again betrayed the many conflicting roles (clinical, managerial, public health, etc.) that GPs play. They discussed its practicability, the ways in which the practice team and computer system could assist or hinder the execution and recording of the new protocol, the acceptability of variations between it and their own varied routines, their own experience of patients, the level at which the new protocol might improve remuneration as well as provide high-quality care, and comparisons with other well-regarded practices (either local or on the internet) that they had found out about.

As a result of such discussions, another partner told us, the agreed ways to practise become 'ingrained I think on my brain to be a good protocol and I suppose what these meetings are doing is reinforcing the good practice. So although we're not actually going line by line through the protocols we're going over the things that we really think are important and that actually forms the basis of the protocol . . . ' But of course there is rarely anything as concrete as a written 'protocol', and even if such a thing exists (mainly to satisfy administrative requirements), it is, as he hints here, not really what matters in day-to-day practice. What matters is the collective view, developed and shared by the Community of Practice, of an appropriate set of mindlines.

Collective mindlines

Throughout the dialogues we have observed, clinicians appear both to be contributing to a joint view of how best to practise, but also drawing upon it. The discussion always allows the participants not only to help mould what we have called 'collective mindlines' but also to adapt aspects of them to their own practice, so that the collective and individual mindlines mutually shape each other. As long as the practitioners then keep within the evolving consensual boundaries of that collective view, they can vary in the way they interpret their own mindlines and implement them flexibly in different patients. Collective mindlines are discussed and jointly understood by the whole group and make explicit the norms of appropriate practice. Like individual mindlines, they are complex, flexible routines for practice that are built up from a mixture of sources melded by time and experience and which are not (and probably could not be) made explicit in the form of a simple written guideline let alone protocol. Indeed only certain aspects of the collective mindline are discussed explicitly. The rest, which is uncontroversial and/or deeply ingrained in each individual, appears to be taken as read. (There is no need to discuss the need to check blood pressure in a hypertensive patient, but there may be discussion about how often the check should be made and by whom and how to ensure that the record is entered correctly in the computer system, and what departures from the norm are within acceptable limits.) The only difference between the individual and the collective mindline is that the latter is the subject of a (largely tacit) agreement to try and conform as a group and is more explicit about putting boundaries around what the group considers to be acceptable practice. Naturally, each doctor tends to vary it a little, to revert at least partly to his or her individual mindline and also to implement it flexibly depending on the circumstances. That, after all, is a key feature of mindlines. The bounded flexibility of the collective mindline always leaves room for the individual to use 'common sense'. Yet the very commonality of that sense – the overlapping of the individual and the collective mindlines – is continually being checked and validated by the social process we have described in the CoP.

There is a variable relationship between individual and collective mindlines. Once the clinicians had thrashed out their views about patients with a marginally reduced eGFR, the GP with the lead for kidney disease (and also for diabetes) told us that there was surprisingly uniform practice in Lawndale. But, he added, 'Targets seem to have changed so much over recent years with diabetes so there's quite a difference between the different aged GPs and what they've been used to in the past. But since this [kidney disease protocol] is new we all started off at the same level.' In our terms, what he seemed to be saying was that it had been comparatively easy to forge a collective mindline of a relatively rare condition whose treatment had not changed very much over the years and where there was not much pre-existing variation in individual mindlines. But for a common disease whose definition and complex management regimes had evolved quite markedly over the years, each GP was coming to the discussion with a different mindline build up over a different period of exposure to the frequently changing received view. In such a case, any collectively agreed mindline would have much more limited overlap with each GP's individual one; the collective template has to be much looser because of the ingrained strength of the differing mindlines that the GPs have each build up over their asynchronous professional careers. In effect, in such a situation the GPs agree the extent to which they can legitimately disagree about some of the details, or put another way, allow looser boundaries around acceptable practice. But if those boundaries are transgressed, then it is understood that the transgressor can be pulled into line, which indeed has happened at Lawndale over diabetes care.

There is a marked contrast between the crisp and concrete statements found in published guidance and the tacitly flexible, evolving, negotiable, virtual, nature of collective mindlines. Yet virtual though collective mindlines might be, they are manifested through tangible entities that can then inform practice, e.g. computerised prompts, instructions to staff, set procedures such as investigation routines, and individual clinical practice and hence outcomes. Collective mindlines formulated by a CoP can therefore be a powerful force in shaping not only patient care but even the perceived existence and nature of the diseases in question. Take the vexed question of deciding the eGFR threshold for treating someone as having kidney disease, which almost all the guidance stated should be an eGFR of 60 or less (see p. 54). As they tussled at practice meetings over the questionable validity and consequences of this guidance, the clinicians over a period of a few months gradually clarified, compared, balanced and reformulated who and what would count as a case of kidney disease. They were negotiating their own individual and collective norms of practice with those advocated by central guidance in order to arrive at the high degree of consensus that had so pleasantly surprised the partner who led on kidney disease. And the conclusion mattered. As a result of the balance of forces in that discussion, hundreds of patients in Woodsea who according to the central guidance might have been identified, labelled and managed as cases of kidney disease ended up not being so. And judging from the similarly unexpectedly low prevalence figures later circulated from GP contract data in 2006, most other practices in the country had concluded likewise. The organisational contingencies of practice were shaping the recorded prevalence of kidney disease not only in Woodsea but also in the country as a whole. The very 'disease' itself was arguably being negotiated into and out of existence.

One might add that the processes that we have described have enabled clinicians collectively not only to come up to date about the management of kidney disease, but, whilst taking due account of the impetus for change that the new contract and guidelines represented, to reaffirm their professional right to treat the condition as they see fit. Arguably, the social development of collective mindlines has given clinicians relatively safe control – and perhaps even a political lever – over what might otherwise prove an overwhelming burden of new knowledge and potentially conflict-ridden demands.

Conclusions

Summary

From our ethnography we have been able to describe several key aspects of the way good GPs may acquire and use knowledge in practice. In summary, they carry most of their knowledge in their heads in the form of flexible, mainly tacit mindlines that have been built up over years of training and experience. Unlike written guidelines, these mindlines, which often rely on 'fuzzy logic', provide immediate guidance in handling many imponderable contingencies of practice that the GPs' multiple roles and varied patients demand. The GPs scan many varied sources, using shortcuts wherever they can to glean information about possible amendments that may need to be melded into their mindlines. They are reluctant to alter those mindlines unless respected colleagues provide sufficient confirmation to do so. They use their networks to ascertain which the most trustworthy sources are. Their immediate colleagues form – at least in our case study – one or more loosely overlapping CoPs that are the first port of call for sharing experience, implicitly comparing mindlines, and testing out new ideas they have gleaned, usually through stories and anecdotes. Unlike most other sources of knowledge, the CoPs share an understanding of *practical and practicable* knowledge that fits their organisational circumstances and roles. Other sources of knowledge – from written guidelines to local hospital specialists to promotional literature – are regarded with caution until discussed among the CoP and brought into a collective mindline held by that group. The collective mindline, which is the local touchstone for practice norms, provides a flexible, bounded, implicit template against which individual mindlines are modified. The mutual influence of individual and collective mindlines happens within the CoP. As a rule only the relevant aspects of collective mindlines – where a change is mooted – are talked about explicitly. The collective mindline provides implicitly accepted boundaries of practice within the group whilst leaving scope for individual variation. This socially based process of the constant crafting and reformulating of mindlines seems particularly well suited to resolving the shifting requirements that shape the way GPs can practise as professionals, and also for handling potential information overload. As a result, both knowledge (e.g. concepts of a disease and its management) and practice (and hence clinical outcomes) can and do change. Also as a result of that process, the GPs assert control over who they are and what they do as professionals.

A CoP and its professional capital

How do these findings relate to the discussion of the model of CoPs and professional capital set out in the introduction to this book? When Lave and Wenger (1991) introduced the concept of CoP, it was in the context of the way people learn. In Lawndale, the GPs are doing a great deal of their learning – or at least improving their knowledge in practice – through their interactions with their colleagues. The group shares many of the features of a Community of Practice as set out in Chapter 1. We see the following:

- **membership** continuing and developing, especially in the multidisciplinary Community of Practice centred on the contract meetings;
- shared **commitment** to improve practice (and succeed in maximising income to the practice);
- an agenda that has much more internal **relevance** to (multi-roled) daily practice than most other educational sources and is also externally relevant to Lawndale's needs as an organisation;
- friendly **enthusiasm** for interaction aimed at pragmatic learning, including a growing energy at the meetings, based not least on the infrastructures;
- **infrastructures** that are very effectively used, including formal and informal communication and ready access to trusted external information;
- **skills** in terms of, e.g. the clinical knowledge skills that all participants bring, the ability to go and find and appraise new knowledge as required from written, electronic and personal contact; and the managerial skill to ensure that once the group arrived at a conclusion, it is usually followed up and implemented organisationally as well as impacting on individual practice;
- Lawndale's **resources** being used systematically to ensure that this happens.

To use Wenger's terms (Wenger, 1998), this is social activity in which learning occurs as a result of the practice staff engaging mutually and sharing a clear understanding of the nature of their enterprise with all its multiple conflicting complexities (which most other sources of knowledge do not share). The participants possess a wide range of shared repertoires (e.g. their vocabulary, their computer routines, their knowledge of the patients and the local services). There is rapid and easy flow of information, often through stories. Through their interactions they negotiate new shared meanings for the problems they deal with, which can entail the reification of practice routines, artefacts (e.g. pop up computer screens or new investigation routines) or even, as we saw in the example of chronic kidney disease, of the perceived prevalence of clinical conditions. (Is a patient becoming labelled with kidney failure a reified artefact of the CoP?) The members of the group develop and reinforce their identity as competent practitioners within their given context; not only do all their contributions demonstrate their value to Lawndale, but membership of the Lawndale CoP improves their own professional positions. By ensuring that Lawndale is renowned as one of the very best practices in the area, they also raise their individual standing among colleagues, health service managers and patients.

The participants learn and develop their knowledge in practice, adapting it to the ever-changing circumstance of the NHS and medical progress. This involves them having to negotiate the terms of what Wenger (1998) would call their 'shared enterprise' (terms such as the right to decide for themselves how they will deal with patients, rather than be dictated to by the Department of Health). The new meanings that they give to the components of their clinical practice (e.g. which patients need what kind of follow-up and why) are deeply interlinked with their continuing need to evolve in order to remain competent and independent clinicians, and those links are fostered by their interactions as a CoP. Their knowledge in practice evolves through the 'shared histories of learning' that come from those interactions. And although we have not discussed it here, Lawndale demonstrates other features that Wenger describes in CoPs, e.g. the admission of new members like trainees and new partners as 'legitimate peripheral participants' who gradually adopt a more central role in their CoP; and the group occasionally excludes those not deemed of sufficient calibre to remain. And finally, although we have mentioned it only in passing, the group members also belong to other communities (e.g. local and national committees, working groups and societies) that allow cross boundary flows of knowledge that Wenger describes.

This CoP also demonstrates many resources that can be called their professional capital, such as the *knowledge and skills*. The clinicians each have their accumulated individual mindlines build over many years of training and experience that equip them to do their job. In terms of the *sociocultural practices*, the groups have not only their collective mindlines, but their shared values and ethos, their agreed ways of behaving, practising and communicating, and their shared history of learning. As 'social beings' they have their *formal and informal networks* of colleagues, along with an acute and subtle knowledge of their strengths and weaknesses. They themselves have the respect and status that they have built up within those networks – especially their immediate colleagues; this enables them to be contributing members of the CoP, which in turn contributes further to their local professional standing. They have the benefits of being part of a dialogue that allows them access to the collective mindlines and the *written and unwritten rules*, which in turn allows them to improve their own professional prowess. And all of these seem to a greater or lesser extent to be dependent upon their membership of CoP.

We set out on this study because the literature on knowledge management had led us to wonder whether part of the frustrations experienced by the evidence-based practice movement might result from having ignored the 'social life' of clinical knowledge. Not only has that view been amply borne out, but the way in which we found the CoP operating may be a pointer to helping to improve the uptake of new knowledge into practice. Until we understand more about the ways in which the CoPs impact upon the development and evolution of clinical mindlines, naïve attempts to introduce new knowledge directly into clinical practice will continue to founder on the rocks of social behaviour.

Methodological postscript

Our ethnography set out to describe the day-to-day activities of a primary care practice, focusing on how clinicians used knowledge in their interactions with patients and carers, and with their colleagues. Our hope was to find key areas where they were formulating changes in their policy so that we could follow how those changes were actually brought about. We expected these to include not only modifications, small and large, in the way clinicians treat patients, but also how they reacted to the plethora of central guidance, not to say pressure, to change the way primary care is organised and delivered. These, we hoped, would allow us to explore the ways in which different sources of knowledge and evidence – e.g. new treatments or research findings, new guidance, or changes in local or national NHS policy – might be put into practice.

These may seem rather heavy questions to lay upon one study of one set of clinicians, but ethnographic research has to trade off the breadth provided by, say, a survey or a series of case studies against the narrower but potentially more profound insights achieved from studying one location in great depth, 'small places, large issues' as one author has tellingly phrased it (Eriksen, 2001). We did consider looking at several GP practices, but in the end we were persuaded that the best approach was to concentrate on one site and then briefly to check out our findings by observing a different, contrasting practice. For our main ethnography, we reasoned that we needed a straightforward practice (not, e.g., academics) but one that practised high-quality medicine, since that would be where we were most likely to see how good clinicians keep up to date and make use of the various available sources of knowledge, including scientific and other evidence. Such top-quality practitioners might be a useful exemplar for others who would like to improve their knowledge management to help raise their standards. Moreover, if we found that in managing their knowledge successfully they do indeed use more complex social processes than the simple linear, rationalistic methods promulgated by the evidence-based practice movement, then we might have important lessons to help mitigate the movement's frustrations.

All ethnographers bring with them some underlying theoretical framework, and it will be clear that we were no exception. Our previous work and our reading of the literature had not only raised in our minds the possibility that we would find clinicians' knowledge to be highly dependent on their social and organisational milieu or, for example, to entail a large tacit component, but also that CoPs may play a part in the way their knowledge was acquired, adapted and used. So even though we had no idea what in this situation such CoPs might look like, nor how they might operate, we needed nevertheless to constantly reflect that the very act of posing our questions with such assumptions might affect the way we saw things. (And indeed, as we have suggested in the main body of the paper, we were so successful in doing so that we failed to appreciate the role of the CoP for well over a year!) We also, like all good ethnographers, needed to be reflexive about the values and cultural assumptions that we brought to our participant observations. Ethnographers need to maintain a crucial balance between getting close enough to the culture to really understand what is happening and remaining distant enough to remain detached. Both of us, having originally trained as clinicians, had been members of the 'tribes' we were proposing to study. So we knew that it would be very easy to get close to the practitioners, but we also knew that we would have to be particularly careful to see their practice with fresh eyes rather than slipping back into the mindset of doctor or nurse. We would need, in other words, to be extra cautious about 'going native'.

We started at Lawndale in 2001 with participant and non-participant observation of around 7 days' worth of GP surgeries, home visits and nursing clinics during which we would briefly explore wherever possible – either immediately or later in more convenient informal settings – why the clinician believed he or she had acted in particular ways. Such exchanges were helped by the fact that we, the ethnographers, were both clinically trained. We also began attending various types of practice meetings (nearly 50 to date) and holding innumerable unstructured informal individual and group interviews and chats. We noted our findings during (or immediately following) our observations or conversations. (Some early meetings and interviews were taped, but we abandoned this as an inefficient method for most of what we needed.) Where appropriate we supplemented our field notes by reviewing written work such as the relevant NHS documentation (e.g. about the Quality Practice Award and the GP contract), practice literature, circulars, professional magazines and guidelines. All of this has taken place intermittently over a period of 6 years, during which we have come to know the practice very well, becoming almost 'part of the furniture'. Since 2003 our data gathering, which still continues now in 2008, has been confined chiefly to non-participant and occasional participant observation of the monthly practice meetings (between 1.5 and 3 hours long), two major visitations at which the practice was being assessed by the Royal College of GPs and by the Primary Care Trust, three educational meetings and about 12 communal coffee breaks in the library, observing – and joining – the general chat. To see if Lawndale was in any way highly atypical, in the autumn of 2001, we also did field work (three surgeries, a practice meeting, three semi-structured informal one-to-one interviews, several short discussions with the GPs and occasional email contact) in a very different practice, 'Urbchester'. This was a highly regarded inner city, university-linked practice in the north of England, dealing with a high proportion of unemployed and immigrant patients as well as students.

The principal analysis used our field notes from the observations and informal interviews, which included detailed observations both about individual clinical encounters and collective formal and informal policy-making. At first we transferred each relevant statement in the field notes and interview transcripts onto around 500 'Post-it' notes and clustered these into emerging themes. Our analysis was informed by several theoretical frameworks rather than being a simple induction. We were, for example, mindful of the role of social and organisational context in the construction and use of knowledge (Callon, 1986; Latour, 1987; Bourdieu, 1990; Berg & Mol, 1998; Mol, 2002), of collective sense making (Weick, 1995, 2001), and of the role of CoPs in knowledge management (Lave & Wenger, 1991; Wenger, 1998). However, we were not testing any hypothesis or preconceived models. As we went along, we noted incidents atypical of our emerging model and used these to test and develop the analysis.

That initial analysis led us to our notion of 'mindlines'. For our subsequent analysis, we discussed after each of the meetings we attended what seemed to be the main emerging themes and subsequently independently read several times through all our recent field notes of the meetings to date, marking out the themes and categories of events and exchanges that we had observed. We critically shared, reviewed and developed the analysis, and as we began to write up the work we undertook specific observations and interviews to check our emerging themes. To help validate our analysis, we tested the credibility and face validity of our findings with the participants at our main study site – a technique often used in such research. But maybe the best 'reality check' has been not so much the affirmations from Lawndale nor the similarity of the picture at Urbchester, but the way so many other clinicians who have heard or read about our study have recognised the picture that emerged.

Chapter 6

LEARNING NURSING IN THE WORKPLACE COMMUNITY: THE GENERATION OF PROFESSIONAL CAPITAL

Mary Gobbi

Introduction

This chapter explores the connections between learning, working and professional communities in nursing. It draws on experiences and research in nursing practice and education, where not only do isolated professionals learn as a result of their actions for patients and others, but those professionals are part of a community whose associated networks enable learning to occur. Several characteristics of this professional community are shared with those found in Communities of Practice (CoPs) (Lave & Wenger, 1991; Wenger, 1998), but the balance and importance of many elements can differ. For instance, whilst Lave and Wenger (1991) describe many aspects of situated learning in CoPs that apply to nurses, their model is of little help in understanding the ways in which other professions as well as patients/clients and carers influence the development of nursing practice. Therefore, I shall argue that it is not just the Community of *Practice* that we need to consider.

At the heart of any discussion of communities and practice lie concepts associated with interpersonal relationships, the moral being and the purpose of community, the knowledge that is explicitly and implicitly communicated within a given community, and thorny discussions about what constitutes practice, theory and action. To attempt to address all of these components in a single chapter would be unrealistic, so I focus on the characteristics of communities of professionals, learning in professional workplaces, the professional capital that is generated, acquired and maintained as a result of that learning, and its relationship to CoPs.

Throughout the chapter I use vignettes from nursing practice and educational activities to illustrate the complexities of learning in workplace communities. The vignettes include examples drawn from fieldwork notes made as a participant observer on cardiothoracic and palliative care units whilst researching the learning and development of registered nurses, especially their use of intuition, reflection and thinking in practice. Other examples are from ongoing work with students

---

Vignette 6.1

The student [nurse] had a query as to whether a thoracic patient could be rolled onto their side or not. The registered nurse stopped, thought and then went to clarify for herself. She went to get the X-ray, looked at it and then checked with the houseman [intern]. They compared the X-ray with previous ones and discussed the situation; the registered nurse indicated that she wasn't happy to roll the patient. She verbally invited the ward sister's [head nurse] opinion, who agreed with her judgement. The sister then called to members of staff and students who were passing by to 'come and look at this' [meaning the X-ray]. This particular situation was not in the textbooks.

---

learning in simulated hospital environments. The chapter commences with three vignettes from clinical practice that raise questions about the nature of CoPs, professional capital and the effects of linguistic and paralinguistic practices.

In Vignette 6.1, a student nurse seeks advice from her supervisor. This example indicates not only the particular nature of clinical decisions, but also the discursive manner through which decisions are made and, for others, the potential for learning occurs.

Does this typical example of A seeking a decision from B, who consults with others before a decision is reached, indicate that a CoP existed (see Chapter 1) in the way Wenger (1998) describes? Or rather, is this more an expression of individuals coming together in a team for a moment of decision making that, through leadership, opens the possibility of learning at work not only for those directly involved but also for others in the vicinity? The driver for learning and action is the need to make a decision about patients in their best interests. Is this a temporary CoP or pragmatic communal action where learning happens as a consequence? It is hard to say – just as it is in practice. Without the intervention of the ward sister, knowledge sharing with the local community would not have occurred. Indeed the cycle of learning and decision making arose from uncertainty about what action to take.

The decision required a 'judgement call'. Gadamer (1973, 1993) links the development of judgement with that of 'sensus communis' (the common sense). Judgement is described as a capacity to subsume 'a particular under a universal, recognising something as an example of a rule' (Gadamer, 1993: 31). However in Vignette 6.1, no one could offer the rule, although interpreting an X-ray in the context of the patient's diagnosis would have been guided by some rules. Gadamer (1993: 39) asserts that judgement cannot be learned theoretically 'because no demonstration from concepts is able to guide the application of rules'; rather judgement can only be 'practised from case to case'. The significance is that whilst judgement is about individual cases, albeit influenced by universals, judgement cannot be logically proven and its explanation may present the individual with discourse problems.

Vignette 6.2

The SHO [junior doctor] attempted to put a line [intravenous line into a neck vein] in the neck, so I stayed by his [the patient's] head; I was now caught pragmatically in the middle by accident... By now I was literally trapped up beside the patient, next to the registrar [senior doctor] who was going to position the scope [fibre optic imaging device].... Around the patient [who was very sick], there were plenty of looks that were exchanged between me and the patient, between nurse L and me, and then between the doctors [whose preoccupation with what they were doing led them to be generally unable to converse with the patient]. Nurse S understood it; there was a lot of silent team work going on in the background... the unspoken acknowledgement that it was better for me to be with the patient.

(working with nurse V month 18)

Professional judgements can be between or concerning isolated individuals or may be within groups of people. From Vignette 6.1, we can recognise the following features of learning and actions in groups:

- learning is provoked by a need to make a decision;
- learning and decision making can involve discussion and consultation between members of a working community;
- knowledge gleaned in practice can be shared through leadership;
- situated learning takes place because the answer 'wasn't in a textbook';
- decision making can refer to the tacit presence of the 'other', namely the patient for whom the decision applies.

Vignette 6.2 provides an illustration of how looks and gazes can be used in professional practice between different professionals and to and from the patient. Here I am working in a high-dependency unit with a patient who has begun to deteriorate seriously; the doctors are engaged in both diagnostic and treatment activities.

Vignette 6.2 reveals signs, signifiers and acknowledgement tokens exhibited through linguistic and paralinguistic devices that need to be learned and effectively employed in order to practice successfully. I found that the learning was embedded within experience, through observation, role modelling and perhaps the advice of others. We also see this in Vignette 6.3, where students are working in small groups to manage and respond to the stimuli presented by a computer mannequin 'SIM-MAN' that provides numerous multi-sensory physical outputs, e.g. blood pressure, heart rate and voice/respiratory sounds.

Each vignette offers us some clues about how professional practice incorporates knowing, not knowing (what to do or why) and doing, as well as paralinguistic and

---

Vignette 6.3

Observing the students around the bedside, one can see how some of them haven't yet learnt to manage and place their bodies. Their resting postures are ergonomically strained, their hands are awkward and they don't know where to put themselves in relation to the bed area. In contrast, others automatically move around the bed, control their hands, move equipment and furniture and position themselves to get the best view of the patient and each other. Some observe their mentor and emulate their movements; others seem oblivious to the mentor's actions.

(video observations, November 2006)

---

embodied skills that even include how to comport oneself. As such the vignettes also offer clues as to the nature and content of professional capital for nursing, which we will now explore.

Professional capital

Professional capital can be described in two distinct ways, one economic and one non-economic. From the economic perspective, professional capital is a dimension of human capital and refers to the skills and knowledge, including tacit and embodied knowledge, necessary for the economic growth and development of the profession. In this context, professional capital becomes, for example, associated with longer periods of education or the requirement to maintain the professional capital held by individual practitioners through mandatory updating or evidence of demonstrable and current competence. Specialist knowledge (Leahey, 2006) and knowledge from evidence-based practice (Goldenberg, 2005) develop professional capital in this economic sense, ensuring that the skills and knowledge components of professional capital are used effectively and efficiently.

Professions also contribute to the creation of economic capital through their role in the production of new technology (Iyigun & Owen, 1999) and science. The relationship between medicine and the pharmaceutical industry classically generates this form of economic professional capital. Additionally, professional capital may be exhibited through particular ways of looking, walking and using body language (Exley, 2001). Such embodied knowledge can carry economic professional capital since economic penalty may result if the wrong image is presented. Thus, the economic perspective of professional capital includes both professional knowing and doing and the embodiment of professional practice.

The second approach, the non-economic one, has origins largely associated with values and beliefs. I call this Personal Professional Capital. It is intrinsically associated with the self-concept of the individual professional and their relationship with others and as McGregor (2004) proposes, it can be viewed as a dimension of a person's philosophical well-being. Non-economic professional capital might include the connections, relationships of trust and mutual obligation and common language that are characteristic of a professional community, as suggested by Lesser and Storck (2001) who draw on the work of Nahapiet and Ghoshal (1998) to highlight this aspect of social capital among professions. Clearly, Personal Professional Capital may also be associated with economic benefit, so that, for example, the public recognition of 'good care' has the capacity to bestow not only personal value for the practitioner and kudos for the organisation but also monetary value by attracting clients to centres of good repute.

Communities of professionals

As early as 1957, Goode's (1957) sociological analysis of professions and their development described a profession as a contained community within a larger society. Although such professional communities may have no physical locus, he writes, many are associated with particular places or brand images with which they give themselves a recognisable way of being, whether liminal, virtual, real or imagined. This in turn enables the community to craft an identity that helps it to maintain a relationship with the wider society as well as provide structure to the community itself.

As a consequence members of a professional community, Goode suggests, are bound by their sense of identity, rarely leave, share common values, have acknowledged role definitions that are understood by members and non-members, share a common language only understood partially by non-members, have power exerted over them by the community itself, exist in a community expressed through social rather than physical or geographical limits and produce the next generation socially through their control over the selection of trainees and the form of their socialisation – a socialisation that might include periods of social isolation from the wider community. Here, it would seem, we already find the fundamental ingredients, as described by Lave and Wenger (1991), Brown and Duguid (1991), Wenger (1998) and Lesser and Storck (2001) of a CoP. In addition, one could argue that communities of professionals, by virtue of the way they learn together, develop a distinctive epistemology – their shared way of knowing about their world. As we shall see later (in Figure 6.1), this epistemological dimension of a community of professionals is an important aspect of their professional capital. However, whilst agreeing that commonality is central to the community of professionals and CoPs, it is necessary to explore further the nature of this commonality within CoPs that comprise professionals like nurses.

Society, communities groups and teams

Some time ago Macmurray (1961) argued that any human society is a unity of persons and that such unity is more than fact, it is a matter of intention. The society

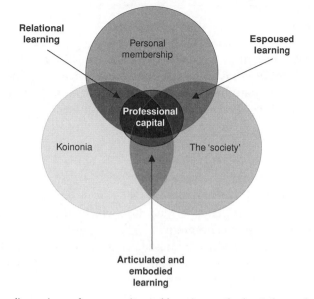

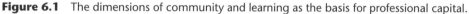

Figure 6.1 The dimensions of community and learning as the basis for professional capital.

remains for as long as its members intend to maintain it. Furthermore he asserts, any human society is a moral entity whose basis is the 'universal and necessary intention to maintain the personal relations which make the human person and individual and his life a common life' (p. 128). He distinguishes between society and community according to the nature of the bonds between the persons who comprise the group. In society, the bonds of relationship between individuals are impersonal and arise from negative motivation, whereas a community is characterised by bonds based on positive personal motivation. Community members are therefore in communion with one another and are associated through fellowship, by practical transactions and by the way they act in relationship to one another.

In the more positive community-based personal relationships that Macmurray spoke of, there is trust. Individuals can think, feel and act together; people are comfortable being 'themselves', relationships can be more authentic and consequently people enjoy freedom as we have shown in the earlier vignettes. If conflict arises and is not completely resolved through the rebuilding of confidence and trust, the relationships may break down or they may be salvaged through the imposition of agreed, mutual restraint. This restraint, of course, diminishes the freedom to be authentic and caring, resulting in the creation of characteristics more akin to those of a society rather than those of a community.

Communities may then resemble the classical Greek concept of koinonia. Whilst koinonia nowadays has theological connotations of communion and fellowship, its root in community incorporates the concepts of sharing, fellowship, association, partnership and common interest. Typically, koinonia engages with beneficial activity that is optimally non-hierarchical and involves actions towards common altruistic goals. Perhaps those communities – such as communities of professionals

Vignette 6.4

She [the relative] wanted me to sort of reassure HIM and I thought well next time, I'll probably say to the person: 'No, (.) I can't lie for you. I can't answer your query' [laughter]. It's not, not just how you actually deal with the patients; it's their relatives as well [ironic laughter].

(with V month 5)

with a strong sense of mission and vision arising from service or covenant roots – may share these features so that their learning will be orientated towards values and practices that uphold beneficent goals. A community of professionals is therefore a very different kind of entity from a society of professionals. This ontological dimension of a community of professionals – i.e. the essence of what it is to be that community – is another important component of professional capital, which like the epistemological dimension of the community discussed above, we will return to in Figure 6.1.

In relation to the professional practice of nursing, clinical freedom comes with the authority and accountability that is held or accorded to the individual professional by the community of the profession. These professional authorities and accountabilities bring with them duties, responsibilities and obligations which may be recognised through discourse. Edwards and Potter (1992) demonstrate that although people who are discussing accountability can, at one level, assign broad responsibility for the events, at another level they are also concerned with the speaker's own accountability for their practice. The interaction between these two levels is shown to be managed according to the context within which it occurs. Vignette 6.4 provides an example of this.

In this de-contextualized extract, several layers of accountability and belief are perceived and implied through V's account. As speaker, V is stating that 'I can't lie for you'; she indicates that she perceives or experiences contrasting accountabilities (responsibilities) between relatives, patients and herself. Learning in a community is often about appraising oneself against one's own and the community's, the profession's and/or civic society's pre-existing values, beliefs and standards. The emphasis is on the person as a moral, socially responsible and intelligible agent and clearly articulates the community dimension of the Person, whose relation to the Other engenders meaningful action (see Macmurray, 1961; Shotter, 1975). Within the context of reflective practice, of course, the Other may be the referential self – i.e. the inner voice that may arguably be speaking for the community.

As Kirkpatrick (1991) discusses, for Macmurray, community is for the sake of friendship and the full expression of a relationship between people, whereas society is for the sake of protection and presupposes fear being maintained by common constraints, for example the law. It is evident therefore that professional communities have the capacity to oscillate between these two modes with implications for the learning and development of their members, so practitioners need to learn now to be a 'professional friend' as well as being an accredited, legitimate professional. Indeed, a legitimised professional community becomes a 'professional' society by definition because of its associated obligation to uphold the espoused and formalised mores of the profession, as well as the laws of the state as they relate to the profession. There is another way to see this: Sergiovanni (1998) cites Sacks (1997) who argued that where a social *contract* is maintained by promises of reward or threat, a social *covenant* is maintained by loyalty, fidelity, kinship, sense of identity, obligation, duty, responsibility and reciprocity and that different types of communities connect as either social contracts or social covenants. Indeed Bradshaw (1994) has analysed the covenant concept in the context of nursing practice. This also suggests that, besides the epistemological and ontological dimensions of *community* (discussed above), which is based more on covenant than on contract, a community of professionals also entails an element of *society*, a formal structure that the profession must espouse in order to be recognised as such. Again, as we shall see later, the formal espoused aspect of a community of professionals is an important aspect of their professional capital.[1]

The Latin roots of the word community denote 'sameness', 'common or shared by many', 'together' and 'performing services' (munis). These themes resonate with professional practitioners in person-based occupations who perform services with and for people, espouse common values and practice and frequently operate in co-located or virtual small groups, albeit now in more inter-professional and interdisciplinary ways of working. In these communities, practitioners share together their professional woes, experiences, hopes, aspirations, achievements and joys in the context of their interactions with each other, their clients, related co-workers and the other persons who comprise the wider society. In order to achieve their espoused goal of professional recognition or status accorded by the relevant society, novices are required to enter, engage with and participate in these communities whilst achieving any personal goals associated with their intended aims. Furthermore, as Lave and Wenger (1991) noted, what distinguishes some professionals from others is the nature of their relationship with their clients. Analyse, for example, the differences and similarities between nurse and cancer patient, defence lawyer and the accused, engineer and industrial client. Vignette 6.5 demonstrates clearly how the motivational effect of caring for the person leads V to learn how to have the courage of one's convictions and to know how to go and 'get the doctor'.

---

[1] Some readers may see parallels between my usage here of the terms 'koinonia' and 'society', and the widely used sociological concepts of *Gemeincshaft*, which roughly speaking refers to the bonds of kinship and shared values and beliefs, and *Gesellschaft*, the bonds of social relationship that are necessary for social function but only in so far as they serve the individual interest. However, I have chosen to use koinonia and society in order to avoid the connotations of those terms that are unhelpful in the context of a community of professionals.

Vignette 6.5a

You go through on your own, that's right. I was saying I would get her [senior nurse] to back me up before, whereas now I would go and bleep the doctor. I would go and get the doctor. That's the difference, I would go. It's having the courage of your convictions as well.

(interview with V month 36)

This vignette echoes back to a prior developmental state where V sometimes had difficulty operating effectively within teams of professionals due to her clinical inexperience. But she was also unable to read and manage the signs of others and communicate in their professional discourse. In reflecting back to the same incident that occurred in month 4, V states as follows:

Vignette 6.5b

...something in hindsight I'm aware of that was also stopping me then. Two things. Firstly knowing you can use the doctors to help you, actually getting access to them. And secondly, having the confidence to go ...I think the problem was I didn't know how to prepare my case properly.

(V month 15)

This vignette illustrated the learning that has to occur within different teams and communities of professionals, in this case the ability to present information in ways that others cannot ignore. V's Personal Professional Capital therefore not only includes a moral dimension, but is also dependent upon traits like courage, multilingual discourse practices and pragmatic knowledge. Experienced practitioners may be able to elicit information from others and thereby facilitate translation from one discipline to another. In addition, we see V's developmental progress acquired through analysing experiences, her own abilities and the interactions occurring in teams both within and across communities of professionals.

Lesser and Storck (2001) discuss the often-confused distinctions between Communities of Practice and teams and refer to the characteristic differences highlighted by Storck and Hill outlined in the middle two columns of Table 6.1. When analysing these characteristics in the context of professional practice (column 4), it is evident that groups of individuals in practice can exhibit the characteristics of both team and CoP. This challenges us to consider what makes the difference – perhaps leadership (Vignette 6.1), personal commitment (Vignette 6.5) or individuals co-located in time who have the ability to share their embodied practice (Vignette 6.2).

Table 6.1 A comparison of teams, Communities of Practice and professional practice

Feature	Team (after Storck & Hill)	CoP (after Storck & Hill)	Professional practice
Relationships	Organisation assigns roles	Formed around practice	Formed around client and role
Authority	Organisationally determined	Emerge through interaction around expertise	Arises through client expectations as well as those of profession and organisation
Goals	Goals set by those not members of the team	Only responsible to their members	Responsible to clients, profession and team
Reporting processes	Determined by organisation	Develop their own	Develop their own in context

Linguistic problems and discourses of professional practice by communities

We have seen that communities can generate their own sense of 'right and wrong' and thereby shape the individual's moral being. Malikail (2003) discusses how 'many aspects of moral life are a matter of imaginative vision and understanding one's own life by analogy to classic narratives' and, citing Aristotle, how the qualities of character are socio-teleological and relate to life in community. The generation, acquisition, transmission and communication of these common values and narratives can require sophisticated discursive practices. Goodwin (1994), for example, identifies the coding, highlighting, producing and articulating of material representations that enable the professional vision to be constructed. This professional vision is the socially organised ways of seeing and understanding events of the particular group: ways of seeing and understanding that need to be learned. Steier (1991: 167) points out that patterns of tacit knowing 'may get unconcealed in conversations' and that attention to stories may reveal 'social ways of seeing and doing'. Analysis of the vignettes (including those that follow in this section) confirms this way of eliciting and learning the ways of 'seeing and doing' as represented through discourse and the analysis of experience as text.

Several of the vignettes have examples akin to Alice in Wonderland's account of *thinking in chorus*:

Alice thought to herself 'then there's no use in speaking'. The voices didn't join in this time, as she hadn't spoken, but to her great surprise they all *thought* in chorus (I hope you understand what *thinking in chorus* means- for I must confess that I don't). (Lewis Carroll, *Alice in Wonderland*, p. 128)

This idea that one can 'think in chorus' indicates connections between silence, language, transmitted meaning and a socio-emotional way of being. As the vignettes demonstrated, occasionally practitioners (and their patients) may not actually verbalise something, but indicate that they shared the same thought as another person.

Ortega commented with respect to the concept of language that 'each language represents a different equation between manifestations and silences. Each person leaves some things unsaid *in order* to say others. Because *everything* would be unsayable. Hence, the immense difficulty of translation: translation is a matter of saying in a language precisely what that language tends to pass over in silence' (Becker, 1991: 226). Applying this to the discourses of practice and their translation implies that practitioners need to learn the purpose of what is said, what is unsaid and the meaning of silence in particular contexts of practice.

Discourses of practice may contain aspects of the 'sensus communis' (the common sense) in which 'feelings or intuition' have an established 'something' with common significance to the community (Shotter's analysis of Vico, 1993: 54). According to Shotter, Vico's 'common sense' arises from socially shared identities or feelings in which an experience/event/circumstance has generated a shared sense with a subsequent 'imaginative universal'. If we take this further, we can acknowledge that the sensus communis can also generate a variety of shared signs and significations that render visible the invisible – at least to a fellow practitioner. From a psychological perspective, a sense of community can be engendered or fostered through a shared emotional connection and is exemplified in the emotional outpourings witnessed at the death of Princess Diana in 1997. In the world of health care, nurses, other health care workers and patients can experience shared emotional connections that strengthen, or indeed challenge the bonds of community or fellowship. Community therefore can be developed through the emotional bonds and ties of practice.

Shared identity is a central element of the professional community; however, the experiences and knowledge of the professional are increasingly becoming available to, and influenced by, lay people. This exchange will shape professionals' knowing and competence and ultimately their professional capital, which in turn will influence the identity, discourses and meaning of being a particular kind of professional.

I have argued elsewhere (Gobbi, 2005) how, when learning to nurse, students and junior practitioners need to learn how to be bricoleurs, both metaphorically, literally, intellectually and technically. Learning how to convey, read and interpret the plurisensorial signs, signifiers and rules associated with what one practitioner described as the 'unsaid stuff of practice' occurs when the moral, relational, intersubjective and permissible or prohibited interactions of practice are exposed: in other words, the professional capital of nursing.

In some situations it seems inappropriate to verbalise the 'unsaid stuff' as this next example demonstrates (Vignette 6.6). I am accompanying T, a palliative care home nurse visiting a patient with cancer. T, the patient, his wife and I engage in silent acknowledgement tokens and the reading of movements and expressions. It is an incident that most practicing clinicians will identify with, even though, as I have argued above, it may not be possible to articulate verbally this 'feeling in chorus'.

This 'unsaid stuff' may include gazes that transmit messages like 'this patient is going to die,' 'come and help me'. They can involve the use of linguistic devices, one I call the 'it cannot be said device'. This device is used when messages need to be conveyed and for whatever reason, words either cannot be said or they cannot articulate a feeling, thought or sensation, e.g. expressing worry, 'there's something

---

Vignette 6.6

The patient began to talk about how his lower abdomen felt more 'full'. He rubbed his abdomen as he spoke, indicating and saying that he could 'feel things'. There seemed to be an acknowledgement by those present that there was deterioration [without a word being said].

(Field notes with T month 9)

---

wrong with that man' where the purpose of the remark is to alert another practitioner to concerns that cannot be verbalised at the time. Furthermore, as Usher (1992) suggested, not all experiences can be communicated, particularly if one tries to read experience as if it were text. In Vignette 6.7, T reflected upon an occasion when we had worked together within a hospice setting. T outlines the complexity of experience and notes how it is not possible to 'write it all down' and 'learn it all from a book' reminding us of the inadequacy of the written word in the context of professional practice.

Foucault (1972: 27) advised attention to the 'silent murmuring, the inexhaustible speech that animates from within the voice that one hears, (to) re-establish the tiny, invisible text that runs between and sometimes collides with them'. In the collective and individual experiences of practitioners and their clients reside invisible texts, the 'unsaid stuff' that runs in and out of practice as exemplified by these vignettes. The appropriate transmission and interpretation of these 'it cannot be said devices' are essential to those present. Foucault claims that 'there is always a secret origin, so secret and so fundamental that it cannot be grasped itself'. In the world of practice and workplace learning, by applying Foucault's recognition that events have 'movement, spontaneity, and internal dynamism' we can gain insights into the learning and doing of practice by and between individuals as well as within the community. It is also possible to analyse the 'continuities and possibilities' present through the influence of others who may or may not be physically present. These influences may be those of power, knowledge and hegemony or influences of emotion and

---

Vignette 6.7

I think that something like we experienced this morning, it's um- it can't be learnt from a book. You can't put all that goes on this morning, every dynamic of it – you can't put it down in a book and tell people what to do. ... You are not going to be able to articulate it. ... It's about getting to know individuals and getting to know PEOPLE as err en masse [almost whimsical voice]. If you know what I mean?

(Interview with T)

---

motivation as seen in the vignettes. Once again acknowledgement of the tacit and personal knowing reminds us of their inarticulate and unspecifiable elements and concepts like hope, commitment, obligation and responsibility that are fundamental to community interactions (Polanyi, 1958, 1983).

The community, learning and professional capital

In summary, we have seen that communities have three significant dimensions. First there is *personal membership* of the community by individuals, possibly working and learning (as in Vignette 6.1) in small teams, who are developing embodied practice. Second there is the nexus of internal community relationships, which I earlier called *koinonia*, which provides the community with its distinctive but intangible ontological and epistemological form. This is the dimension of the community that gives its individual members the cultural propensity to practise in certain ways, whether alone or collectively, and to adopt communally approved forms of both explicit and tacit knowledge.[2] Third there is the formal dimension of the community that conforms to the notion of *society*, as discussed above. Here we find the formal, contractual and regulatory dimension of the relationships between the individuals that may be the basis of a professional society and its espoused effect on the wider world. Figure 6.1 is an attempt to show how these three dimensions of a community of professionals integrate to generate professional capital.

This integration is achieved through the various types of learning that arise from the different dimensions of the community, which come together to create an active, emergent, and sometimes contested zone in which members generate and utilise their professional capital. More specifically, these types of learning include the following:

- **relational learning** between the individual members, generating and transmitting cultural, 'tribal', informal learning/knowledge and creating embodied action;
- **espoused learning,** which includes the formal and legitimised codes, ethics, practices, semantics and theories of the profession;
- **articulated/embodied learning,** which comprises the repository of collective formal and informal knowledge.

We have seen in the vignettes that the professional capital generated through learning is strongly influenced by professional (un)certainty and moral conviction, and that the learning of a range of linguistic and paralinguistic skills is also crucial. Foucault highlights this necessity 'because it means giving the key of a language that masters the visible' (Foucault, 1973; 114). Visible and invisible aspects of professional practice are exposed in the professional workplace as the medium not only

---

[2] There is a parallel here with Bourdieu's concept of the *habitus*, which he first described in the 1970s, and which is the propensity for members of a culture to act in particular ways that they have learned from each other over a lifetime (Bourdieu, 1990).

through which learning, communication, action and reaction take place, but also through which professional capital is generated.

The centrality of the client in generating professional capital

Learning is also inherently stimulated by the needs of clients, who play a key role in the accumulation of learning and professional practice and hence are vital to the creation of professional capital. Through their interaction and engagement with professionals, they play their part in each dimension of Figure 6.1.

Personal membership of the profession allows each individual to have a personal portfolio of clients with whom they directly, indirectly or vicariously interact, learn about and learn from. This portfolio forms the basis of their professional and personal embodied practice and contributes to their Personal Professional Capital. Because personal membership inevitably results in involvement with the koinonia of specialist networks or communities (in Figure 6.1, this is the intersection of 'personal membership' and 'koinonia'), they share a vicarious client group that gives them much more professional capital through their clients/or their representative user groups than they could ever achieve as individuals. Learning at this intersection is relational and allows the individual (student or qualified) access to the accumulated pool of knowledge from those clients. Depending upon the way the koinonia works, there may be a more or less accessible archive of client experience that is shared informally through such relational learning. Additional knowledge about (or from) clients may come from other professions/disciplines who relate directly to the community.

Moving round to the next dimension in Figure 6.1, membership of the 'society' – the formal, regulatory aspect of the profession – is what gives the professionals direct access to their clients, since, for example, no nurse may treat a patient until s/he is formally licensed to do so. This formal access to clients is also regularised, constrained or augmented by the influence of a range of other stakeholders (for example, doctors, managers or politicians). Individual members of the community must formally engage in the community's espoused learning, mediated, for example, through curricula that delineate the theoretical strategies for interacting with clients. However, much of the formal learning overlaps with, and is mediated by, koinonia, and it is in this intersection that the professional is accorded access to the shared repository of client memories and archives. These may be acquired through many different media, such as individual client stories, the representations of user groups and, increasingly, information from digital repositories and interactive media. This gives the member a far wider repertoire of client experiences than would otherwise be possible.

So far, this chapter has explored aspects of learning and development in professional practice, using nursing as an exemplar. In so doing, it has proposed a view of professional capital that is integrally related to the client, for without the client there can be no meaningful professional capital for nurses. Professional capital may be both visible and invisible to its members and their associated clients or lay community, but it is learned, maintained and developed by professionals through the social practices of their communities.

The relationship between community, CoP and professional capital

Sergiovanni (1998) in the context of US schools has suggested that CoP could be cultivated as a way to generate professional capital as 'a fabric of reciprocal responsibilities and support' (Sergiovanni, 1998: 40) for both the members (i.e. the teachers and the students) and the community institution (school) concerned. Sergiovanni emphasises the importance of communities, the leadership of the communities and the learning that occurs within them. These elements are connected through learning in close proximity to others within a physical and social environment that allows people to focus on matters of importance.

This view is of course transferable to health care and more specifically to nursing where the professional capital associated with nursing is linked not only to the individuals directly involved in care – the nurse and the patient – but also to the impact that good (or poor) nursing care can have on the organisation in which care is provided. In transferring Sergiovanni's model to the health care context, one may see that CoPs could enable nurses to ask questions and learn together and also care together so that they are able to construct professional capital that helps them (and their organisation) navigate through the complex world of nursing. We saw this illustrated, for example, in Vignette 6.1. However, as we also saw in that vignette, and as I have argued above, one does not necessarily need to invoke the concept of a Community of *Practice* (except perhaps as a local subset of the community of professionals) in order to envisage how that team of nurses was able to generate the necessary professional capital.

Lesser and Storck (2001) describe how organisations benefit from CoPs, which have been shown to improve performance through the sharing of knowledge, through bypassing structural barriers by operating outside formal structures, and through their contribution to organisational memory. The communities/teams outlined in Vignettes 6.1, 6.2 and 6.5 show how organisational memory can be developed (1), exist (2) and be invisible to the neophyte (5). We saw how the nurses gained, or had the potential to gain, from using their community as a resource for learning and achievement, but it was also clear that this relied on all the facets of the wider community that I have been discussing.

Leadership of a community involves the mobilisation of the members to face problems, solve them and maintain the espoused standards of both the immediate CoP and the broader community of professionals. Sergiovanni uses the term 'head follower' to reflect the leader's role and obligation with respect to the professional community's ideals, purposes and commitments. It is in this sense that – whether or not it is a CoP – a community of like-minded people functions as a moral community drawing on similar values and ideas and generating professional capital. The reciprocal influence shared by other influential communities may include mutually acknowledged obligations, but this does not always occur – as in Vignette 6.4, where those obligations were neither clear nor shared between the relatives and the nurse.

Professional capital and learning in the workplace community

In this chapter I have argued that learning among professionals operating in groups in the workplace needs to take account of the way they generate, disseminate and acquire professional capital within their community of professionals. Situated learning theory proposed by Lave and Wenger (1991) and Wenger (1998) has contributed significantly to the conceptualisation of learning outside formal educational institutions. Like Fox (2000), Lesser and Storck (2001) and Boud and Middleton (2003), I recognise the value of situated learning, but also that it is not a sufficient explanation of informal workplace and/or organisational learning. This is because situated learning theory focuses largely on cognition, meaning and concepts of identity and does not place sufficient weight on the effects of others, the developmental stage of the practitioner; the moral person and moral community. These factors also influence the decision-making processes, judgements, actions and discretionary practices. Furthermore as we have seen in complex workplaces, there are overlapping communities and the distinction between team, group, CoP and broader communities of professionals may be fluid in the context of the 'here and now' and the needs of clients.

Boud and Middleton (2003) remind us that learning at work comprises a major component of learning undertaken by adults. Theories of how adults are thought to learn and the conditions that foster learning in professional practice include work on learning in and from experience, developmental theories, the role of the organisation itself, socialisation and andragogy. Knowles *et al.* (2005) summarise the core principles of andragogy, namely the importance of a learner's need to know, their tendency for self-directed learning, the role of prior experiences, the person's readiness to learn, their orientation to learning and problem solving and finally their motivation to learn. They conclude however that 'learning is a complex phenomenon that defies description by any one model' (p. 202).

Boud *et al.*'s (1993) analysis of learning through experience outlines five propositions that underpin their work, namely that:

- experience is the foundation of and the stimulation for learning;
- learners actively construct their experience;
- learning is a holistic process;
- learning is socially and culturally constructed; and
- learning is influenced by the socio-emotional context in which it occurs.

Certainly, the vignettes in this chapter support these propositions, but also perhaps suggest that they underplay the importance of communication devices in workplace learning, along with the more widely perceived obligations of the profession and the associated drivers of personhood and moral conviction. Within professional communities, learning is intrinsically related to the nature of the professional's experience as well as the demands of professional competence and the influencing factors of others. Echoing Billett (2002: 4), the vignettes support the view that the 'structuring of experiences in workplaces is often inherently pedagogical [i.e. educational] as they are directed towards the continuity of the practice through participant learning'.

The vignettes suggest that leadership, role modelling, embodied practice/knowledge and professional vision may also be significant influences on both individual and community development and learning. Professional practice demands learning practices that are client focused, embodied, holistic, reflexive and can occur with or without cognition but always involve 'doing now' or envisioning the 'doing next time'. What is evident is that the analysis of professional capital allows us to understand better how that learning is stimulated, enabled, structured, archived, recognised and retrieved in communities of professional practice. Not only client needs but also the needs of the profession dictate that workplace learning for both neophyte and expert will develop and be reflected in nurses' emergent professional capital.

Chapter 7

COMMUNITIES OF PRACTICE AND LEARNING HEALTH PRACTICE IN DEVELOPING COUNTRIES

Alex le May

Introduction

Action on global inequalities in health has been galvanised by international policy initiatives such as the Millennium Development Goals, whilst the broader development agenda has been championed in economically developed countries through a coalition of politicians, non-governmental organisations (NGOs) and well-known cultural figures. Consequently, there is widespread interest and support for improving the livelihoods and health status of the billions of people living in developing countries. Overcoming the extent of ill health is central to the current development agenda. According to World Health Organisation (WHO) estimates, sub-Saharan Africa alone suffers 25% of the world's disease burden despite being home to only around 10% of the world's population (WHO, 2006). Yet the restricted supply of health practitioners available limits the rate of progress in tackling ill health in developing countries.

Recent initiatives at the global level have developed a strategy for training health workers and improving health practice. The limited rate at which traditional health training can be scaled up has stimulated interest in innovatory approaches to learning that seek to make better use of international training resources through the internet. Existing international networks of practitioners have subsequently been strengthened and new networks have formed. This chapter outlines a number of initiatives to build Communities of Practice (CoP) for the learning of health practices in low-income countries. The analytical and practical contribution of the CoP discourse to improving health practice in developing countries is considered.

Health care practice in developing countries

In most developing countries 'modern' health practices, founded on biomedical knowledge, have international origins. European missionaries and colonialists introduced Western practices of hygiene and medicine to Africa, South America and much of Asia in the late nineteenth century. In the European colonies in Africa, medicine arrived to serve the colonisers, rather than the colonised. Early hygiene programmes were introduced to maintain the productivity of key workforces, such as those in plantations. Medical techniques were extended to African populations in the early twentieth century, serving a largely urban population of wealthier Africans and colonial bureaucrats. Large teaching hospitals were built and stocked with advanced medicines and equipment providing similarly advanced standards of care. In the lead-up to independence from Britain, African medical schools were partnered with British ones, producing doctors of equivalent standard to those graduating in Britain. Meanwhile, rural and poorer sections of the African populations had little or no access to medical practices.

During the 1950s and 1960s, the state-backed expansion of medicine continued the trend of training health workers to a high standard, but with skills that bore little relevance to the health needs of the majority of the population. Responding to the inequities of health care practice, the primary health care movement was cast around the Alma Ata declaration of 1978. This landmark convention encouraged innovation in the practice of health work in developing countries, challenging the dominant model of doctor and nurse led provision of health care. Subsequently, the training of community-based health workers with comparatively little medical training was pursued in many developing countries.

Today, practices of health care, health promotion and the management of health services in developing countries are defined within a context of endemic diseases, largely overcome in wealthy countries. Whilst high life expectancy and low morbidity has been achieved with limited national income in some developing countries such as Costa Rica, Sri Lanka and Cuba, the burden of disease in middle- and low-income countries differs markedly in extent and form from that of high-income countries (see Figure 7.1). Many factors account for these global inequalities. Economic, behavioural and ecological factors conspire to create malnourishment, a high rate of infectious diseases such as malaria, diarrhoea, respiratory infections and HIV, alongside a high burden of physical and psychological traumas associated with rapid economic change and conflict. Yet a central reason for the extent of disease in developing countries is the limited capacity of health systems to respond to disease due largely to the limited availability of trained health professionals to provide health promotion and health care services. In sub-Saharan Africa, there are only 2.3 health workers per 1000 population, whilst in Europe the figure is 18.9 per 1000 population (WHO, 2006). Statistics presented in this way, whilst clearly showing inequality between regions or countries, mask unequal access to care within many health systems. In Ethiopia, for example, in 2005, 6% of births were attended by a skilled birth attendant, but among the poorest fifth of the population the figure was only 0.7% which has serious consequences for the safety of women in childbirth (ibid).

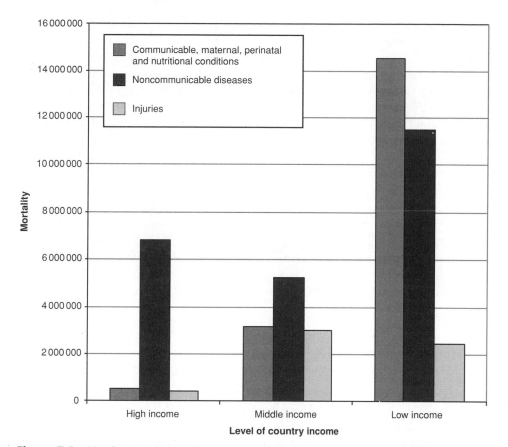

Figure 7.1 Distribution of mortality by disease category and country income level in 2002. Data from: WHO (2004a).

Despite similar disease contexts across many developing countries, one should be cautious when generalising about health practice in these countries. Practice is likely to be shaped by varying political objectives, economic limitations and legal frameworks that guide health systems and the goals of organisations that facilitate health practices within health systems. The role of traditional forms of health practice should not be underplayed. Depending on the symptoms, the extent of illness and the ability to pay, patients often consult both local, and traditional, health practitioners alongside or as opposed to biomedical practitioners. However, broad international trends in economic and social policy have produced certain homogenising trends in health care planning in developing countries. International development and public health organisations have an important role to play in shaping health systems and thereby defining health practice in developing countries. The World Bank and the World Health Organisation have explicitly influenced health systems through stipulating conditions for health sector lending and technical support whilst also encouraging the spread of knowledge about the structure of health systems and their financing.

Through these international organisations, the primacy of state-led health care provision that emphasised doctor-led care has been challenged. In most developing countries today, the state remains an important provider and purchaser of health services, but the ascendance of a free market economic paradigm within international development agencies in the 1980s and 1990s and the fall of the Soviet Union carved out an increasing role for private sector provision across the health systems of developing countries. The increasing plurality of health care provision in developing countries has been intensified by the growth of the 'third sector' or civil society in providing health care; local faith-based health providers, local and international non-governmental organisations and social enterprises have provided an increasing number of health services. Since the 1970s civil society organsations have been strong advocates for radical innovation in health practices, for example, the development of specific practices for vulnerable populations such as sex workers, refugees and women.

Civil society organisations have also been key advocates and providers of community health worker schemes, and many governments have developed national programmes (Berman *et al.*, 1987). These workers are defined as:

> members of the community where they work, who are selected by those communities, who are answerable to those communities for their activities, who are supported by the health system but are not necessarily a part of its organization and have a shorter training than professional workers. (WHO, 1987)

Community health workers are consulted by large sections of the population in many developing countries and engage in a very different kind of practice to their fellow clinic and hospital-based health workers including behaviour change, political mobilisation and monitoring practices. Their activities may also include those ascribed to social workers. Alongside community health workers, NGOs have also often tried to involve health practitioners who specialise in non-biomedical, 'traditional' health practices to deliver services at a low cost to hard-to-reach populations. The proliferation of community health workers and traditional health workers within the health systems of developing countries has added to the range and diversity of health practices.

Expanding health practice in developing countries: The need for innovation in learning methods

The shortage of health workers in developing countries has recently gathered increasing attention. The Global Health Workforce Alliance was founded at the World Health Organisation to coordinate global action and the issue surrounding the shortage of health workers became the central theme in the World Health Report 2006 – *Working Together for Health*. This was also a core concern of a recent report to the UK government (Crisp, 2007). The WHO report identified a threefold strategy to address the shortage of health workers in developing countries: recruiting more health workers, improving the capacities of the current workforce and reducing the number of workers leaving the health care professions in developing countries. Success in the first two elements of the strategy requires that greater attention is paid to innovation in learning if health practice is to be advanced and health improved.

Medical schools and specialist public health training facilities in developing countries are at the forefront of training health students needed to fill the shortfalls in qualified health workers. Cuba's Latin American Medical School draws students from across Latin America, West Africa and even the USA to train as health care providers. Funded largely by grants from the Cuban government, some 22 000 students study medicine in Cuba. The Cuban example is notable because of its significant contribution to training health professionals and spreading health practices in developing countries, not to mention significant innovation in the content of that practice, but health training on this scale does not exist in other developing countries, limiting the current potential of health schools in developing countries to produce sufficient new health staff to fill current shortages.

International solutions have been considered. Many health professionals from developing countries travel to European and American medical and public health schools, often with financial support from their governments and international student bursaries such as those from the Ford Foundation and the Commonwealth Scholarship Programme. Yet, this is clearly not a sustainable solution to the problem of training health workers in sufficient quantities to serve the significant health challenges of developing countries. Consequently, new opportunities for international learning offered by the internet, mobile and satellite communications through a range of teaching and learning techniques are being suggested by health care training organisations under the banner of 'e-learning'. These allow practitioners to learn and share practice without the need to travel great distances and contribute to both the first and second objectives of the WHO's strategy – training more workers and improving the capacities of the current workforce.

Distance learning uses communication technologies to facilitate student–teacher interactions, and to a lesser extent student–student interactions, beyond the classroom. Daniel (1998) traces the origin of distance learning to Saint Paul's letters to the early Christian churches, making the comparison between the priests who interpreted and gave voice to these letters for their congregations to modern-day tutors who facilitate modern-day distance learning. Modern distance learning can be traced back to commercial training courses distributed through the postal service in the USA during the 1950s. This was subsequently developed through a wide range of media in Europe by state-backed academies such as the UK's open university. The principle of distance learning has been adopted by public health schools in developing countries. For example, the London School of Hygiene and Tropical Medicine runs a number of distance learning courses that are marketed globally, whilst the Info Project at the Johns Hopkins Bloomberg School of Public Health in the USA provides students with on-line presentations, reading lists and other learning resources in disease prevention, health promotion and population training via the internet. Specialist networks of medical and nursing schools have emerged to provide virtual medical and nursing education to students in both developed and developing countries, such as the International Virtual Nursing School and International Virtual Medical School, whilst NGOs such as African Medical Research Foundation have developed programmes of distance learning for training health practitioners in developing countries.

Advances in communication technologies are also being proposed as a means of providing information and advice about case-by-case practice between health workers in developing countries and in developed countries or between rural and urban health workers. Telehealth or telemedicine links medical practitioners through the internet and satellite technologies facilitating live consultation between health workers about clinical decisions, and in preventative and managerial practices.

Whilst use of the internet offers health workers the potential to overcome barriers of distance and time to learning new practices, it also offers opportunities to consult with other health practitioners through initiatives such as telemedicine. These rely on the existence of networks between health practitioners or other means of putting health practitioners in contact with one another. Although the technology to communicate across great distances allows consultation and group reflection on practice it relies on relationships being established between practitioners working in the same field of health practice or practitioners being able to access networks of other practitioners with relevant knowledge. Communication technologies are a useful means of bridging distances and time, but social relationships still underpin the potential of these technologies.

Communities of Practice

Communities of Practice refer simultaneously to a theoretical framework that describes a social body, in which learning takes place and explains the learning process within such communities, and a learning model that has been promoted as a means of sharing knowledge between practitioners. It is a relatively new addition to the vocabulary of managers, practitioners and academics working to improve health in developing countries, and for many the term is an unknown and perhaps confusing piece of management jargon that could easily be overlooked. The notion of CoPs may also provide an analytical tool for the exploration of the relationships that underpin the learning of practice between health practitioners and as a model for improving learning. Indeed the model has been embraced and analysed to some extent by a number of major development and public health institutions – notably those based in North America. The World Bank's Knowledge Management function – the World Bank Institute – runs numerous Communities of Practice, including a number within the field of health, that bring practitioners and academics from both within the World Bank and its partners together around a shared topic of interest. A number of initiatives from within NGOs and the broader civil society have also adopted the Communities of Practice framework.

The conceptual roots of the term *Communities of Practice* lie in Jean Lave and Etienne Wenger's (1991) book *Situated Learning: Legitimate Peripheral Participation*. Focusing on the integration of newcomers into a workplace, Lave and Wenger developed a theoretical account of learning that outlined the process by which a newcomer is initiated into a set of practices within a workplace. Workers or practitioners learn much of their practice 'on the job' from colleagues in spontaneous groups or communities that emerge in the workplace. This learning occurs through observation and participation in the day-to-day practice of the community and reflection on the group's work and their working environment(s). The notion of Communities of Practice was then further developed by Wenger (1998) in his analysis of ethnographic accounts of the North American workplace, which resulted in building theories of workplace-based learning from his observations. Since its inception, the notion has come full circle from a critical exposition of the limited validity of managerial accounts of learning in the workplace to becoming a 'tool' that managers might use to embark on better knowledge management.

Originally Lave and Wenger (1991) proposed that communities emerge in situ, where learners are based within close proximity and are constantly interacting with one another. In contrast with traditional didactic learning, characterised by a hierarchical relationship between expert teacher and student in which the expert teacher imparts knowledge to a group of students, learners in a CoP learn from their fellow community members through informal conversation about their practice or observation of one another's practice. It therefore suggests a more egalitarian and dynamic set of pedagogical relationships. Alongside the practices involved in getting a job done, Communities of Practice are contexts for the formation of professional identities among the community's membership. Communities of Practice, and the identities that are developing within the communities, reproduce themselves through the practice being passed on to new members when they join a group – a theme explored in detail by Wenger (1998).

Brown and Duguid (1991) proposed a subtly different notion of a Community of Practice to Lave and Wenger's (1991) earlier analysis through their synthesis of Orr's ethnographic accounts of service technicians solving problems. Orr showed that instead of seeking a solution from some form of abstracted guidelines such as their organisation's repair manual – this they term 'canonical learning' – technicians solved problems by eliciting advice about similar problems in the form of narrative accounts from their colleagues and then drawing lessons from these stories to apply to their particular situation. When dealing with a problem, technicians seek this support from their most immediate, trusted colleagues which for Brown and Duguid is synonymous with a Community of Practice.

Although there are subtle differences in observations, Brown and Duguid's account of CoP is, in several ways, very similar to that of Lave and Wenger (1991). Primarily they share the finding that learning takes place through groups of close friends or colleagues. This process of learning is also contrasted with 'orthodox' approaches of didactic or canonical learning in industrial economies. Brown and Duguid retain Lave and Wenger's assertion that CoPs are necessarily constituted by a local membership. However, the outcomes identified by Brown and Duguid differ as a CoP is seen to be of interest to organisations as a means of solving problems, rather than the locus and process of identity development for its members proposed by Lave and Wenger.

Perhaps the most influential text on CoP outside academic anthropology and organisational science is Wenger *et al.*'s (2002) *Cultivating Communities of Practice*. This widely cited text approaches CoPs as a potential tool for managers to use for enhancing learning to meet workplace objectives. Although the empirical evidence presented in this book is less rigorous than in earlier texts, the book offers a far more accessible entry to thinking about CoP. Here they offer a definition that is all encompassing and represents – for me – a significant shift from earlier concepts. Communities of Practice are:

> Groups of people who share a concern, set of problems, or a passion about a topic, and who deepen their knowledge and expertise in this area by interacting on an ongoing basis. (Wenger *et al.*, 2002: 4)

Instead of referring to practice – a central concern in academic anthropology given its role in the formation of individual and collective identity – a CoP refers to a group who share 'a common concern, set of problems, or passion about a topic'. This could include anybody from any professional background; a group of people without a linking professional background working within an organisation; people from a number of organisations or a group of people not working within an organisation at all. Instead of working side by side, most likely for the same organisation, members of a CoP only need to interact on 'an ongoing basis' to satisfy the membership requirements of a CoP as now laid out by Wenger *et al.*, they need not necessarily be located near to one another.

The notion of a CoP now seems to have moved from a necessarily intra-organisational, localised and professionally homogenous group of colleagues who are probably also friends, or enjoy high levels of trust for one another, to an ideal type of a looser social group in which people are tied together by little more than a common interest and their ongoing interaction. Although this shift seems to place less emphasis on the role that CoPs have in the formation of the identities of their members, it is not entirely lost in the later, looser definition. Members are likely to join because they have already established a professional identity and seek to share knowledge with similar self-identifying practitioners. Whilst this conceptual shift fuels a good deal of the confusion associated with the terminology and calls into question the use of the word 'community', which often refers to groups that interact within close proximity to one another having already established some collective identity, it may also offer greater opportunity for using CoPs for learning health practice in low-income countries where health communities are widely dispersed.

Communities of Practice for enhancing health practice in developing countries

The broad conceptual status of the CoP makes an analysis of international CoPs in health practice conceivable. Indeed the terminology and learning models espoused in the literature on CoPs have been explicitly adopted by international development organisations. If members who join a CoP because they share 'a common concern, set of problems, or passion about a topic' do not need to reside near to one another and interact face-to-face, they could therefore be spread across the world, interacting through the internet or telephone. Consequently, some organisations have adopted the CoPs terminology, whilst others have organised programmes that develop relationships between practitioners through which learning about health practice can take place, bringing groups of health practitioners working in both wealthy and developing countries together to share knowledge garnered from their various activities. It is possible, by using the CoPs framework, to identify three kinds of international CoPs that address the learning needs of health systems in developing countries: intra-organisational, inter-organisational and inter-practitioner CoPs.

The extent to which the CoPs analytical framework and/or learning model has been used within organisations that seek to improve health practice in developing countries is difficult to gauge. Organisations are unlikely to have the time to document the practice or analyse the impact that using a CoP framework is having when compared to other approaches; indeed they may not even use the CoP tag to label learning programmes or their analysis of learning. However, one case study has been documented by Ramaswamy *et al.* (2005), who outline the adoption of the CoPs framework for improving organisational learning within the American humanitarian NGO Care International. Care managed to successfully adopt the CoP learning model across a highly compartmentalised and international organisation. They demonstrated the applicability of CoPs within a development organisation and its impact on practice. Other similar documented examples are difficult to find, but it seems safe to assume that an analysis of learning within international health care organisations or within in-country state, private or civil society providers would find other examples of CoPs.

NGOs and development agencies frequently work in partnership with one another on specific health programmes. Much of the work of development involves the facilitation of partnerships between health service delivery organisations in various countries, thereby bringing health practitioners from across the world into contact with others and allowing relationships to emerge across organisations. Through these relationships, information about health practice can be shared between practitioners – examples of this can be seen across Europe. For instance, the French government's work promoting and funding links between French hospitals and those in the francophone developing world. The Portuguese-speaking countries have also developed a network of activities, including linking organisations to support developing countries to improve the health of their populations. In the UK, the Links Programme, facilitated by the Tropical Health and Education Trust (THET) seeks to develop lasting links between health-providing organisations in the UK and developing countries to facilitate the reciprocal transfer of knowledge and skills between partner institutions. These programmes involve managers, clinicians, academic staff, non-clinical staff, support staff and students enabling international communities of health practitioners to emerge across organisations, lasting beyond the exit of core members from the community.

A brief browse on the internet will bring users into contact with a number of on-line or 'virtual communities.' One example, the Implementing Best Practices (IBP) Knowledge Gateway Initiative run by the IBP Secretariat at WHO's Reproductive Health and Research Division and the INFO Project at Johns Hopkins Bloomberg School of Public Health, is an interactive forum through which policy-makers, programme managers, implementing organisations and providers convene to identify and apply evidence-based practices that can improve reproductive health outcomes in their countries. The website has a membership of 4300 practitioners from 132 countries who participate in 56 communities, with membership within each community ranging from 10 to 1200 people. These communities can pull on a broader membership than intra- or inter-organisational CoP. Members potentially have access to a network of health practitioners of global proportions who can provide knowledge and experience from a wide range of types of health practice and health practice contexts that can serve narrower knowledge requirements of specific health practitioners. These inter-professional communities are less likely to be constrained by the strategic direction of an organisation or a formal inter-organisational partnership that may determine the range and extent of practice-related knowledge among community members in intra- or inter-organisational CoP.

Concluding comments

The development of CoPs that are international and often virtual raises a number of practical and analytical issues. The following section identifies some of these issues and whilst it is not a systematic attempt at evaluating international CoP, it does provide a medium for raising some of the merits and limitations associated with trying to build CoPs for health practice learning between health practitioners across developed and developing countries. The main themes identified here are the barriers posed by access to the communication technologies that facilitate international CoPs, the notion 'community', and the potential for learning through relationships across great distances. In addition, the applicability of the CoPs framework – developed in North America – to learning in low-income countries is considered.

The internet and other forms of new communications are cheap and much desired goods in developing countries. Developing countries have been identified as emerging markets by internet providers and mobile phone operators; yet despite high demand and expanding supply, the internet is still not widespread and is frequently of low density, suitable only for text and not images. Computers are not robust and maintenance is difficult. Internet access is within reach of between 20 and 40% of most African nations, whilst in the US around 87% of the population are able to access the internet (WHO, 2004b). The Crisp report cites an unpublished paper, prepared for the Global Health Workforce Alliance, that shows that even where there is a wide range of information and communication technology (ITC) facilities available – paper, phone, fax, video, email, discs and DVDs – there is still a tendency to make most use of the most traditional means (Crisp, 2007: 148).

Barriers to access will be felt particularly acutely at the lower levels of care hierarchies in developing countries, i.e. for nurses and community health workers. Community health workers have the potential to gain considerable information to support their practice from the internet, but they are often located in remote areas with poor access to the internet and even in areas where the internet is supplied they are likely to have such low incomes that voluntary consultation of colleagues on a regular basis through the internet is impossible because of lack of funds. It is therefore likely that accessing virtual CoPs and other internet-based networks or communities of practitioners is more realistic for programme managers, policy-makers and the better educated and wealthier cadres of health workers than it is for lower-level front-line health workers.

Using the term *Communities of Practice* to describe particular groups of learners is a useful rhetorical means of putting people at ease and making them more willing to relax any possessiveness towards 'their' knowledge. Community is a warm term that supposes trusting relationships between well-meaning individuals and could be a welcoming 'brand' for networks of learners that require their members to enter into relations with trusting states of mind. However, this is a new addition to the language of health practitioners, and therefore the concept and the learning model espoused requires explanation if it is not to be dismissed.

The word 'community' has connotations of a group of people living locally, interacting in person regularly. Lave and Wenger's original notion is explicit about the local nature of community. Does this mean that a CoP should be local? Practitioners will have differing preferences for the level of face-to-face interaction and rapport they seek to build with others in sharing practice. In fact, some practitioners are likely to prefer to learn from people with whom they have only a superficial, internet-based relationship; however, it should be remembered that a recent review of the literature on virtual CoPs found that a number of evaluative studies noted the importance of face-to-face contact, especially to build an initial rapport (Johnson, 2001). This suggests that there are limitations on international, virtual Communities of Practice, in which resource constraints limit the opportunities for face-to-face interaction. Practitioners will find it hard to build strong and trusting relationships with practitioners who they rarely – or never – interact with in person, thereby perhaps needing to imagine themselves as being part of a community.

Perhaps the most important issue in applying the CoPs framework to low-income settings is the generalisability of the framework and model across the cultural and economic divide between high- and low-income countries. The CoPs framework was developed in North America. Subsequently, using the learning model drawn from this framework to facilitate learning among health practitioners in low-income countries and between health practitioners across the world relies on some compatibility between the features of social learning in North America and that in say Uganda, Burkina Faso or Nepal. Sensitivity to the cultural differences between North America, or other nations of the 'western world', and low-income countries is required in the application of the CoPs framework and learning model. Furthermore, within low-income countries regional and ethnic variations make it very difficult to generalise about learning and about practice with certain practitioners being better resourced and more inclined to 'intercultural' communication than others.

An important next step in the application of the CoPs approach to low-income countries is therefore to return to the earlier concern of the CoPs paradigm – an exploratory analysis of social learning. Exploring the ways in which social learning occurs in low-income countries is an important stage in the growth process if low-income countries are to become better able to harness the potential for sharing practice and learning not only locally but also across the borders of international CoPs. This sort of exploration will provide critical knowledge about whether the CoPs framework has the potential to foster greater, more appropriate and effective learning across the different communities of people who provide health care in developing countries.

Chapter 8

GENERATING PATIENT CAPITAL: THE CONTRIBUTION OF STORYTELLING IN COMMUNITIES OF PRACTICE DESIGNED TO DEVELOP OLDER PEOPLE'S SERVICES

Andrée le May

Introduction

This chapter examines how storytelling evolved as a mechanism for exposing lay knowledge and integrating it with professional knowledge in three Communities of Practice (CoPs) working towards the development of older people's services in one Strategic Health Authority in England. The research work that this chapter is based on was both developmental and evaluative aiming both to construct and develop the CoPs and to describe and evaluate their workings; we did not explicitly set out to study storytelling. Rather we became interested in it as our analysis revealed its centrality to enabling the CoPs to integrate professional and lay knowledge. The chapter's structure reflects the natural process of the research.

Background

Involving people who use health and social care services in the design, development and evaluation of these services has, over the last 15 years, become an increasingly important focus for both central and local UK government policy-makers. The NHS Plan (Department of Health (DH), 2000) and subsequently the National Service Frameworks (NSF) have situated patient representation clearly at the centre of modernising health and social services by promoting more involvement from citizens (i.e. actual/potential clients/patients and carers) in the design, development and evaluation of services. The centrality of this proposition to current UK health and social policy has therefore resulted not only in policy-makers and health and social care professionals placing greater value on lay knowledge but also the increased use of this type of knowledge (or evidence) in service design, development and evaluation.

Recent policy in the UK spells out the importance of lay knowledge in the creation of patient/client-centred services. This is evidenced particularly in relation to (1) the management of illness and chronic diseases (Expert Patient; DH, 2002); (2) the evaluation of people's experiences of health and social care through satisfaction surveys at both local and national levels (e.g. National Patient Surveys, and others carried out by the Picker Institute [www.pickereurope.org]) and complaint monitoring through the Patient Advocacy and Liaison Services (PALS) and Commission for Social Care Inspection (CSCI) as well as through other specialist advocacy services (e.g. for mental health) and ombudsmen; and (3) the design and development of services through involving service users either locally (e.g. through local implementation groups linked to the National Service Frameworks or patient involvement forums and networks associated with the Commission for Patient and Public Involvement in Health (CPPIH) or Local Involvement Networks (LINks)) or nationally (e.g. through the CPPIH or membership of national patient representative organisations and listening/consultation exercises [e.g. About our health, our care, our say; DH, 2005b]).

In order to support increased patient and public involvement, there has been a proliferation of training opportunities, literature and 'tool-kits' to help both professionals and citizens involved in such activities to do so more competently and confidently. These include the public engagement toolkit (NHS Executive, Northern and Yorkshire, 1999) aimed at primary care services, the establishment of the patient and public involvement programme by the Public Health Resource Unit in Oxford (2002/3) to enable professional and lay participants to work as partners on health concerns and more recently the production of role play games (e.g. Trust me I'm a patient; DH, 2004) designed to promote better involvement of patients and the public in service changes. There has also been an emphasis on raising the profile of patients' experiences, e.g. through a wide-ranging internet-accessed database of patients' experiences (DIPEx, www.dipex.org) and promoting greater collaboration between patients and health care professionals rather than the more traditional approach in which the patient is seen as a passive recipient of care (Coulter, 2006).

One group often perceived as under-represented in health and social care consultations is older people (le May, 1998). However, specific attention has recently been focused on involving older people more in the design, development and evaluation of local services (including health and social care provision) through, for example, the 'Better Government for Older People' (BGOP) initiative (Cabinet Office, 1998), the ongoing work associated with the NSF for Older People (DH, 2001) and the work involved in the Partnerships for Older People Projects (POPP) (DH, 2006b).

The central drive towards explicitly valuing and using lay knowledge has several benefits related to the improvement of services and the development of a greater understanding between lay and professional groups, as well as the growth of a user-friendly, supportive evidence base (Cayton, 2004). But some may still perceive it as undermining traditional evidence hierarchies that give primacy to research and generalisability rather than experiential knowledge, and professional rather than lay knowledge. Stacey (1994: 89) writing close to the start of the evidence-based practice movement in the UK contrasted professional and lay knowledge (or as she called it, 'people' knowledge) stating that the latter comprised knowledge gained from past experiences; in the case of consumers of health care services, this was a mix of old medical knowledge and knowledge acquired through being part of an existing health-related experience. Lay knowledge is characterised as complex, experiential and – because it is rarely taught or codified in books – passed on informally by word of mouth; professional knowledge on the other hand is systematised, generalised and more likely to be associated with formal learning (Stacey, 1994). She goes on to warn that the perceived differences (and currency) of lay and professional knowledge may, when service users and providers work together, result in power struggles and the need to 'put lay understanding and lay experience into official language' (p. 91). One of the challenges for service development is therefore to find ways in which the two types of knowledge can be ascertained and merged in order to develop patient/public informed services. One solution is to work with patients seeing them as experts and partners in the process of health and social care delivery as the National Institute of Health and Clinical Excellence (NICE) and the Social Care Institute for Excellence (SCIE) in England and Wales are doing; another solution may be to design multi-agency, multi-professional CoPs with strong patient/client representation.

Fully embracing the movement towards greater citizen involvement means going beyond what is often viewed as the conventional professional–patient encounter characterised by the consultation or by canvassing patient opinion via questionnaires, interviews or focus groups and moving towards, for example, a more integrated approach in which health, social care and voluntary sector workers, patient/client representatives and citizens work and learn simultaneously together to communicate and use a variety of types of knowledge in the design, development and/or evaluation of services. This type of approach challenges the traditional interface between the health and social care sectors and the public (either individual citizens or those patient/client organisations who represent them). One of the main challenges is finding a common language, not just at the obvious level of avoiding exclusive terminology but at the deeper level of finding a mutually comprehensible mode of discourse that can allow different types of knowledge a fair voice.

This chapter examines how older people's services were developed through the integration of professional and lay knowledge in three CoPs clustered within one Strategic Health Authority in England. Communities of Practice are increasingly being recognised as a key to learning and practice development in a wide range of organisations (e.g. Bate & Robert, 2002; Wenger, 2006). This chapter describes the ways in which a range of health, social care and voluntary sector workers, representatives from patient organisations and citizens came together with a view to designing and developing new services for older people around single assessment, intermediate care and services for impaired hearing, and how storytelling emerged as a vehicle for exchanging knowledge in the CoPs.

The research design

Three CoPs were developed during the course of two research studies (Lathlean & le May, 2002; Gabbay *et al.*, 2003) that aimed to explore the ways in which CoPs might improve local health and social care services for older people and how knowledge flowed within them. Both studies used similar methods in order to:

(1) construct and develop the CoPs (focus groups with citizens and professionals were used to identify topics for consideration and initial membership of the CoPs; the subsequent CoP meetings were facilitated by two members of each research team in order to help the CoP to develop services);
(2) describe their workings (non-participant observation and tape recordings of CoP meetings were made by two researcher/evaluators, semi-structured interviews of CoP participants focusing on their experiences of being in the CoPs and their use of knowledge were also undertaken by the researcher/evaluators; the facilitators and the researcher/evaluators each wrote reflective diaries).

Data generated from these techniques are summarised in Box 8.1. Details of the facilitation and workings of the CoPs are presented elsewhere (Gabbay *et al.*, 2003).

The CoPs comprised lay persons with a shared interest in being involved in developing services for older people (via BGOP or patient representative organisations) and health and social care workers from the NHS, local authority social services and housing departments, the voluntary sector and the private sector (see Boxes 8.2 and 8.3 for details of the range of groups represented). Each CoP met seven times with

---

Box 8.1 Sources of data

CoP meetings

CoP notes generated from flip charts and acetates used by the facilitators during each meeting. These were circulated to members together with other relevant attachments (published papers, reports (local and national), web pages and letters between CoP members).

Observation notes and tape recordings of each CoP meeting made by researchers.

Interviews with CoP participants
Recordings of semi-structured interview.

Reflective accounts
Kept by the two facilitators and the four researcher/evaluators.

Box 8.2 The range of groups represented by participants in the CoPs, focusing on single assessment and intermediate care

Local citizens
Community health council
Citizen's advice bureau
DISCASS (disabled citizens' advice and support services)
Red Cross
Age concern
Primary care group(s) (chief executive and general practitioners)
Community trust (nurses, physiotherapist, occupational therapists)
Acute trust (nurses)
Residential/nursing homes sector (physician)
Health authority (planner)
Social services (social worker, discharge coordinator)
Housing department (manager)

Box 8.3 The range of groups represented in the CoP, focusing on hearing

Local citizen representative and service user
Primary care group (purchaser)
Primary health care (general practitioner and practice nurse)
Acute trust audiology services (consultant)
Acute trust ear nose and throat services (ENT) (medical consultant)
Social services (occupational therapist)

attendance numbers varying from 5 to 15 participants as the project progressed and participants co-opted others to attend the meetings.

The results

The data (Box 8.1) were merged and analysed thematically for each CoP to expose the variety of types of knowledge used by the CoP (Boxes 8.4–8.6). As part of this analysis the research teams asked two questions:

- What features appear to foster working together?
- What features appear to hinder working together?

Box 8.4 Types and sources of knowledge identified in the single assessment CoP (examples)

Types of knowledge	Sources of knowledge
Lay perspectives	CHC and BGOP representatives on CoP National Patient Survey
Discharge information and patient information sheets from acute and community services	Local trusts
Studies/research on how people cope	King's Fund
Work from elsewhere	King's Fund, Central Middlesex Hospital, Sheffield Project
Local policies	Single point of access to occupational therapy scheme
Audits of re-admissions	Trusts
Stories	CoP members

In answering these questions, it became clear that stories, told spontaneously (eliciting stories was not a technique deliberately used by either of the facilitators), were a key way in which knowledge was exchanged in the CoPs and fostered working together within them. (Other features of knowledge transfer and utilisation have been explored elsewhere (see Gabbay *et al.*, 2003)).

Box 8.5 Types and sources of knowledge identified in the intermediate care CoP (examples)

Types of knowledge	Sources of knowledge
Experiences of people using rehabilitation services	Local survey of rehabilitation (2001); CHC
Patients' needs	Local GPs and nurses
Studies of intermediate care	King's Fund
Local provision of intermediate care (including voluntary sector, local authority – what boundaries exist) and evaluation of schemes Evidence of effectiveness	Joint investment plan (JIP), citizen's advice bureau, charities, social services; health authority (director of public health), meals-on-wheels (borough council), intermediate care coordinator, community trust, acute trust – discharge team; good neighbour scheme
Stories	CoP members

Box 8.6 Types and sources of knowledge identified in the hearing CoP (examples)

Types of knowledge	Sources of knowledge
Professional opinion	Experts in ENT, health service commissioning, social services provision of services of people with sensory deficits, general practice and speech and language therapy within CoP
Patient/client experiences Patient/client needs	Patient perceptions (one participant also described her work with older people and their views on hearing)
Policy documents	Guide to integrating community equipment – Department of Health Stepping away from the edge – social services inspectorate RNID best practice standards for audiology services (draft)
Evidence of effectiveness through empirical work	Health technology assessment review related to community provision of NHS hearing aids and related audiology services for adults RNID report – audiology in crisis – still waiting to hear NICE guidance on hearing aid technology Fully equipped – audit commission report
Stories	CoP members

The stories were all 'historical narratives or anecdotes' (Shorter Oxford Dictionary, 1973) primarily concerned with the realities of care. They were often short, sometimes stemming spontaneously from discussions of another source of knowledge being examined (e.g. a research report); at other times they were irrelevant to the specific topic covered – rather they emphasised a deeply held perspective of a CoP member often linked to personal experience of health and social care services – for instance, local hospital closures or car parking inadequacies at health centres. Despite the haphazard way in which they were used in the CoPs' discussions, they provided an effective mechanism for sharing knowledge across the membership of the CoPs.

The stories could be grouped into three main types each having a different purpose. The first group related specifically to firsthand experiences of services, the second gave voice to the experiences of others and the third was a mechanism through which different sources of knowledge were integrated.

Stories of firsthand experiences of good or poor practice/inadequate services

These stories and their telling tended to dominate the first meetings of the CoPs, helping members to establish their place in and likely contribution to the CoP by showcasing their knowledge about the services on which the CoP was to focus its work. Storytelling at this early stage of the CoPs' development allowed members to contribute, and interpret relevant knowledge, without being intimidated by professional jargon or boundaries, and in that way to begin to set down the foundations of each CoP's knowledge base. The storytelling activity itself appeared to break down barriers allowing each person an insight into the other's world, providing a means through which members could ease their way into the CoP and gain credibility (or not) within it. This was particularly so if they were not already 'known' to other members of the CoP or in an authoritative position outside the CoP, e.g. within the local health and social care community (as for instance were the chief executive of the Primary Care Trust, a local medical consultant/general practitioner, etc.).

This type of story – one in which care was exposed and described – also allowed CoP members to experience, albeit vicariously, realms of practice that were unfamiliar to them, e.g. doctors gained insight into the professional worlds of, for instance, voluntary sector workers or the lay worlds of older people managing to care for dependent relatives when they themselves required professional care; older people were exposed to the complexities of managing health service budgets and balancing the needs of the wider population against the individual's. The storytelling also provided on rare occasions an opportunity for members to vent anger at local service provision – in one extreme example a lay member wrote accounts of problems she and her family experienced locally and pointedly read them out to the CoP. Most reacted sympathetically and politely, but a manager/clinician from one of the 'accused' organisations was motivated to provide documentary evidence of the procedures and policies used to guide practice; even in this case the knowledge base of the CoP increased.

Stories giving voice to the collective experience of others

These stories provided an opportunity for CoP members to extend the knowledge of the CoP by giving voice to other's experiences from outside the CoP. This provided more knowledge for the CoPs which was, on occasions, translated into concerns for the CoP to focus on. For example, in the hearing CoP the patient representative, in response to questions from the facilitator, told a number of stories about hearing loss that reflected the experiences of a group of senior citizens that she belonged to. She concluded by saying that 'hearing loss means they are alone and trapped'. She then used these stories as a means of identifying needs and types of services required.

In the single assessment CoP, one lay member similarly brought knowledge from outside to the CoP. She had surveyed her friends about keeping their own medical records in their homes for all visiting professionals to use. She recounted the findings of her survey in a narrative form creating a graphically illustrated story of her friends' fears of patient held records – for instance, the cleaner might read sensitive information not only about the care that the person was receiving but also about other social and financial circumstances, and this may become a source of local gossip and embarrassment. This story was then used by the CoP to back up research findings which had been presented at a previous meeting; together the research and the story as an alternative source of evidence provided a powerful argument which persuaded the CoP to move away from patient held records – they were never mentioned again.

Stories giving voice to CoP member's experiences in response to the presentation of other sources of knowledge in the CoP

In addition to the story of the survey that supported research findings in the single assessment CoP, we also noticed the use of stories in the intermediate care CoP to help make the research findings more meaningful. Such stories usually spun out of a discussion of a research paper. In one example a group of CoP members was detailing the findings from a systematic review of evidence for the CoP to consider. Part way through the description, one professional member of the CoP started to tell a story about when he was a practitioner which was sparked by the discussion of the systematic review. This led to another member taking up the conversation with another story of their practice. The information from all of these sources (although relatively incomplete) was then synthesised by the CoP into a way that care should be delivered in the local community (Gabbay *et al.*, 2003). The findings from the systematic review were discarded and forgotten, but the stories that resulted from it gained prominence and contributed to the CoP's decision making.

All of these stories appeared to help each of the CoPs to understand more completely the service area selected for improvement by providing accounts of various elements of the services, either as providers or as users of them, thereby creating a history of services experienced by older people and their professional and non-professional carers. In doing this they enabled the CoP to function in the ways described earlier in this book by Wenger *et al.* (2001: 4) and formed a mechanism through which knowledge was shared and deepened through interactions and patient capital increased. For instance, stories stemming from the presentation of other sources of knowledge in the CoP helped the CoPs to draw together and meld knowledge from research, practice and local experience allowing them to situate the unfamiliar research within a more recognisable reality of their local practices. On occasions the stories also opened up opportunities for the service providers to explain why certain things were happening – for instance, why the local hospital was short of beds for people convalescing or why independent nursing homes could not provide the numbers of beds that NHS/social care managers needed.

Although the stories were told by all members of the CoP, thereby giving voice to both lay and professional experiences, they were always told in a lay rather than professional or 'official' voice and as such could be easily assimilated into the working knowledge of the CoPs.

Discussion

Whilst storytelling is an everyday occurrence, it has only recently gained credibility as a way of eliciting knowledge about health and illness (e.g. Greenhalgh, 1999), exploring organisational life (e.g. Czarniawska, 1997) and implementing change in organisational practices (e.g. Llewellyn, 2001; Bate, 2004; Seely Brown *et al.*, 2005). Little attention has been paid to its potential as a means of sharing knowledge in intergenerational, multi-agency, multidisciplinary groups developing and/or redesigning health and social care services. Existing reviews of storytelling in older age focus on its potential for promoting intergenerational understanding and sense-making of old age (e.g. Hepworth, 2000) or on it being a mechanism for negotiating and sharing the meaning of being old among older people – thereby encouraging group cohesion through the sharing of written and oral stories – fictional (e.g. in poems and novels), biographical or autobiographical (Jerrome, 1992).

Although we did hear stories that explicitly linked the older participants in the CoP providing greater coherence and thereby 'voice' for them, the majority of the stories extended intergenerational understanding enabling the sharing of knowledge across the CoP rather than divisively among subgroups of the CoP members. This was achieved through the use of lay language in the stories and their use to transform what could be described as problems experienced individually into public issues (Gibson, 2006) for the CoPs to work with. Closer examination of this process reveals a number of facets.

Firstly, the stories provided a framework for participants to make sense of the multiplicity of views and experiences expressed. The stories were, as Warner (1994: xi) suggests, like material artefacts in museum displays which 'reveal ways of life, interest and activities, social arrangements;' and in so doing exposed the members of the CoPs to the several communities that each represented. For example, the geographical community in which a range of services (e.g. intermediate care, single assessment) was to be provided; the community of service providers who experienced the difficulties of caring within, for instance, resource and skills constraints; the community experiencing the consequences of growing older, e.g. a 'hard of hearing' community, a community in which help from others was an integral part of maintaining independence, a community within which personal information was made public, a community in which multiple assessments led to confusion and disorientation rather than clarity about the care being provided. The academic literature, fiction and autobiographical material teem with examples of each of these communities, but these writings lack the immediacy offered by the stories told in the CoPs. Telling and hearing them firsthand enabled the CoPs to take the stories, work with them by exploring different viewpoints from within the CoP, meld them with evidence from research or other developments across the UK and then provide solutions in terms of models for service development for the CoP to work with and disseminate beyond the boundaries of the CoP.

Secondly, the stories told by (or on behalf of) the older members of the CoPs gave meaning to the experiences of health and illness so that they could be construed by the other members of the CoPs. This enabled the CoPs to consider how services could be constructed in order to preserve or restore health or support a reduced level of health and ongoing social functioning. These stories brought to life the lay perspectives of health and illness in older age found in the literature (e.g. Herzlich, 1973; Blaxter, 1983; Calnan, 1987; Williams, 1990). The stories showed how older people managed their own health and well-being in the context of their everyday lives. They reinforced the importance of health at a personal level through the absence of active disease, and if this was not possible the management of disease so that a balanced life characterised by positive well-being and social involvement could be achieved.

Thirdly, some of the stories of personal experiences of services were used to augment or make real the data presented from the research studies and/or policy documents that the CoPs examined. Like Polanyi (1985), who suggests that this linking of stories to some prior comment may make them more enduring, we noted that this melding of different types of knowledge opened up conversation in the CoPs and thereby increased participation and debate. The stories then allowed participants to feel that they could contribute to the knowledge base of the CoP by engaging in day-to-day communication rather than having to rely solely on more advanced skills in information retrieval or appraisal. This gave value to members' contributions increasing not only the knowledge capital but also the social capital of the CoPs (Seely Brown, 2005).

Fourthly, we watched a storytelling etiquette develop within the CoPs, one in which everyone's story was listened to even if it was not always acted upon. This resulted in the CoPs achieving many of the applications that Denning (2005b: 177) describes in relation to storytelling in organisations such as the ability to communicate complex ideas effectively and efficiently, the development of a sense of involvement and the ability to persuade others to change.

Finally, the stories were used by the CoPs to seed, beyond their boundaries, organisational change in the NHS (Denning, 2005a; b) resulting for two of the CoPs in their lay members being co-opted onto NSF local implementation groups focusing on single assessment and intermediate care, allowing the patient capital generated in these CoPs to be reinvested in another influential forum.

Conclusions

There has been a tendency to dismiss stories, often labelled 'anecdotes', as the worst form of evidence, even to the extent that they have become anathema to the evidence-based practice movement. But our findings among the three CoPs revealed this to be an oversimplified reaction that underplays their important role in conveying information and generating knowledge. Of course, like all other sources of evidence, such stories need to be 'critically appraised' but to ignore them altogether would be to throw the baby out with the bathwater. Telling stories in these CoPs enabled members to hear the voices of patients and service users, sometimes from the periphery before they mastered techniques for moving to take the centre stage, sometimes from its core as they gained confidence and credibility within the group. Accomplishing this through the lens of the recipient, not just the professional practitioner or policy-maker, allowed the CoP to have a better understanding of how services were perceived and received as well as wanted. And conversely, it was often stories told by the service providers that helped the lay members of the CoPs to understand the organisational problems that needed to be overcome. Each set of stories helped the CoPs to decide what was needed in order to improve care and to ultimately design services better for the people using and working in them.

The lay members of the CoPs developed strategies for telling their stories as the projects progressed. Some were successful; the survey of friends, for instance, collected and presented information in ways familiar to the professionals so had immediate credibility (the fact that the storyteller also handed out slices of her homemade cake was not the deciding factor in whether the information was used by the CoP – but it did help to create the all important 'social fabric of learning' (Wenger, 1996) within the CoP). Others were not so successful: the long catalogue of relatives' woes that had been so pointedly read out to the group was never used again.

The patient capital generated by these CoPs did not have to compete with professional capital – in fact, in most instances, the two were readily merged. This worked positively for the CoPs, and although it is not possible to attribute this ease of merger directly to the use of storytelling as a technique for integrating patient and professional capital, it is possible to suggest that storytelling, because of its inclusivity – everyone can take part in it, either as teller or listener – does have the potential for not only generating patient capital but also helping to merge patient and professional capital in health and social care.

Part 4
SO WHAT?

The earlier chapters have shown quite clearly some of the advantages and limitations of Communities of Practice (CoPs). The last part of this book tempts readers to think about the impact, or potential impact, of CoPs in health and social care. In Chapter 9, Helen Roberts, Alan Shiell and Madeleine Stevens challenge us to use Communities of Practice as a means of commenting on and influencing what works, what counts and what matters in health and social care.

The final chapter allows me to ask the real 'so what?' question – where does this get us and where will we go from here?

WHAT WORKS, WHAT COUNTS AND WHAT MATTERS? COMMUNITIES OF PRACTICE AS A LOCUS FOR CONTRIBUTING TO RESOURCE ALLOCATION DECISIONS

Helen Roberts, Alan Shiell and Madeleine Stevens

Background and introduction

Health, social care, criminal justice and education are all areas of service provision where the resources available in any society are unlikely ever to meet demand. Whilst those of us who work in the public sector understand this, the principles of social justice which have traditionally underpinned the welfare state in the UK can frequently make the subject of resource allocation uncomfortable. Those whose task it is to inform (let alone carry out) resource allocation are sometimes portrayed as remote, heartless and penny-pinching, knowing the price of everything but the value of nothing.

In this chapter, we suggest that mechanisms which attempt to allocate scarce resources openly and transparently are likely to be preferable to other kinds of systems, which might, for instance, depend on the ability to argue one's case well, or being fortunate enough to have a teacher, social worker, nurse, doctor or youth justice worker who will do so. If one of the purposes of welfare provision in the UK is to make effective 'treatments' available to all, free at the point of access, it is important to bear in mind the potential of different systems of resource allocation to widen, rather than narrow, inequalities. Assessments of cost-effectiveness are not, therefore, an alternative to social justice but a means of pursuing it.

In order to know whether a particular intervention or policy is cost-effective, we first need to know whether it is effective – in other words, does it 'work'? We therefore start by describing some of the work of our ESRC-funded What Works for Children project (www.whatworksforchildren.org.uk), which ran from 2001 to 2005, and aimed to put research evidence into the hands of practitioners and planners, and respond to their expressed needs (including requests for data on costs).

We go on to describe work currently in progress looking at, and appraising, cost-effectiveness analyses for the same 'nuggets' of evidence on which we had earlier searched for cost data.

We then say something about the extent to which practitioners in different disciplines and professions are exposed to literature which considers costs, cost benefits and cost-effectiveness, and what this might mean. This leads us into some of the background to resource allocation in the UK in one area of scarcity – health – and we draw in what we say below on some of the mechanisms used by the National Institute for Health and Clinical Excellence (NICE) in England and Wales.

Given the importance of cost-effectiveness, it seems to us that there is a need to consider how the evidence is received locally – how it is interpreted, whether it can be translated, and what happens when the evidence is incomplete, contested or does not appear to be a good 'fit' with local priorities. We therefore conclude by starting to explore whether Communities of Practice (CoPs) might play a greater part in informing, as well as responding to, resource allocation decisions in social care.

Bringing research and practitioners closer together

'What works?' is a fundamental question for policy-makers, practitioners and service users. As well as asking what works, and how to implement it, we also need to think about what does not work, and how to stop it. For those of us working on the What Works for Children initiative, improving outcomes for children is not just a research, policy and practice issue for those of us at the supply end. It is also a rights issue for those on the receiving end of services. Moreover, the question of the best return on a society's investment in human services through taxation is a crucial one, whether it relates to services delivered at an individual level or right across a population. Social, criminal justice, health and educational interventions are often complex and capable of doing as much or even more harm than medical ones. The What Works for Children project worked predominantly at the implementation end of the evidence agenda, with our work and our project outputs designed for those whose task it is to plan and deliver services. We built on a body of work demonstrating that research is not readily available to practitioners in child public health, particularly social care and nursing, that even if available, it may not be useful, and even if useful, it may not be used as the result of a range of barriers (Barnardo's Research and Development, 2000; Brocklehurst & Liabo, 2004). We worked in partnership with the UK's largest children's NGO, Barnardo's. Our questions were as follows:

- How to make research findings available to those who provide or manage services?
- How to make the available research meaningful?
- How to get meaningful research into practice?

The resources we produced with and for our Barnardo's partners (and freely available from the website) included an evidence guide, now expanded and updated by Barnardo's (Frost *et al.*, 2005), a project planning and review tool, research briefings and overviews, and a review of practitioners' priorities on the basis of not only our own, but also others' surveys (Stevens *et al.*, 2007). Questions of cost-effectiveness did not come up explicitly in the review of practitioners' priorities, though practitioners did identify as a priority issue:

Funding: lack of it, how to manage with insufficient funds, where to get funding

Taking note of the evidence from the research utilisation literature, we also set up an evidence-request service in order to support social care practitioners in using research findings in their service planning. An implementation officer within Barnardo's worked with service planners to identify areas where research could be helpful. Researchers, meanwhile, provided responses to practitioners' questions by searching for, critically appraising and summarising the relevant literature (Stevens *et al.*, 2005). This service found a degree of mismatch between practitioners' needs and available research. Gaps identified included information on costs of interventions, on implementation, and on interventions carried out in a UK context. We also produced 'evidence nuggets', summaries of sound evidence which we put out to practitioners from whom we had sought advice on content, length and the kinds of information they needed. Practitioners asked for information on costs for planning purposes. Service planners and practitioners were interested in data on costs which might be helpful in making a case for a particular intervention. It is important to make the distinction here between wanting information on costs for planning purposes and wanting cost-effectiveness data. In the former, a decision has been made to try and implement something and the cost data is used to support the case for funds. In the latter, the evidence on cost effectiveness, for example, what outcomes one could expect to achieve at what cost, informs the decision about whether or not to implement an intervention.

Box 9.1 shows some of the information that we were able to retrieve in one of our nuggets in relation to costs.

The kind of data in Box 9.1 on costs alone is, of course, rather thin, and our current work, funded through a small grant from the Nuffield Foundation (Stevens *et al.*, 2008) is to explore the extent to which there is related economic evidence to support (or otherwise) the cost-effectiveness of interventions we describe in our evidence nuggets and to look at the kinds of outcome measures used, i.e. what is measured as an indicator of success? Box 9.2 gives an example of a current issue demonstrating why outcomes matter. Where there are economic studies, we are reviewing their quality using a validated measure (Chiou *et al.*, 2003) and considering the problems that might arise in using the evidence locally (Sculpher *et al.*, 2004; Arai *et al.*, 2005), something to which we return in our final section.

Box 9.1 One-to-one mentoring programmes and problem behaviour in adolescence.

Mentoring programmes have been targeted at groups of children experiencing difficulty in their lives as a result of their challenging behaviour; for example, those referred by schools, police, court, social welfare agencies (Grossman & Tierney, 1998; Tierney *et al.*, 2000); identified as having multiple and serious difficulties (e.g. contact with police and history of exclusion) (Tarling *et al.*, 2001); pregnancy whilst still at school (Havens *et al.*, 1997) or with diagnosable behaviour problems (St James-Roberts & Samlal Singh, 2001). Young people in these difficult situations are often brought into contact with welfare agencies in the hope that early support may offset later disadvantages.

The main costs of mentoring programmes are in managing the scheme and providing training and support for mentors who are usually volunteers from the local community. The recruitment, training and matching of mentors and young people demand significant resources. In most schemes care has been taken to match the mentor and mentee for gender, ethnicity or experience. The aim of this matching is to increase the likelihood of successful relationships forming, although research has not supported this theory (Du Bois *et al.*, 2002).

The Dalston youth project provided educational support and a residential weekend as well as mentoring. Total running costs were £110 000 per year. On average 19 young people were recruited to the project per year, making the average cost per young person £5800. Had the maximum of 30 young people completed the programme, the cost would have been £3700 (Tarling *et al.*, 2001). Project CHANCE cost approximately £10 000 per child per year during the 1997–2000 evaluation period, although again the projected cost was lower (£3000 per child) based on an estimate of larger numbers of children completing (St James-Roberts & Samlal Singh, 2001). A study of the cost of 52 mentoring programmes in the USA found that the average budget was $324 000 per programme and $1114 per mentee. The range between the programmes was wide, from an average of $12 to $1900 per young person per year. When including in-kind donations and the voluntary work (mainly provided by the mentors), these figures increased and no mentoring scheme was able to provide services for less than $189 per young person, with some costs as high as $9000 per mentee. The larger programmes had higher costs (Fountain & Arbreton, 1999). We do not know whether this is because larger programmes require more paid administrative work or whether they provide more-intensive mentoring.

(www.whatworksforchildren.org.uk/docs/Nuggets/pdfs/Mentoring%20nugget.pdf)

> **Box 9.2** Is investment in drug treatments worthwhile?
>
> The BBC Radio 4 Today programme on 30 October 2007 reported on the amount of extra funding going into drug treatment services in England – a budget increase of £130 million since 2004–2005. However, over this period, only an extra 70 people were reported as having been weaned off drugs – a cost, as the commentator suggests – of £1.85 million for every addict drug free at the end of treatment. But of course, our view of the value of this intervention depends on what 'counts' as an outcome. If effective treatment means being drug free, then the intervention does not look promising. If it includes cutting crime, generally improving health, supporting families, and so on (and if, of course, the treatment succeeds in doing this), then it may not be quite such a disastrous investment.

Practitioners' exposure to resource, cost and cost-effectiveness issues

Whilst there can be no public sector manager or practitioner who is not exposed daily to the realities of budgets, costs and resources, to date, much of the work in social care, education and youth justice has been on costs, or allocation of resources, rather than the kinds of cost-effectiveness studies seen in the health sector.

There are, however, some good examples of cost-effectiveness research. One important trial which looked at the issue of cost-effectiveness of a complex social intervention is the Perry High/Scope study, an early childhood education programme. It has been calculated that for every $1 originally invested in this programme, there has been a return to the taxpayer of over $7 in real terms as a result of reduced crime, lower demand for special education, welfare and other public services (Barnett, 1993). In brief, by the age of 27, graduates of the High/Scope pre-school programme had significantly higher monthly earnings (29% vs 7% earning $2000 or more per month); a significantly higher percentage of home ownership (36% vs 13%); a significantly higher level of schooling completed (71% vs 54% completing 12th grade or higher); a significantly lower percentage receiving social services at some time in the last 10 years (59% vs 80%) and significantly few arrests (7% vs 35% with 5 or more) than those who had not been randomised to the intervention (Schweinhart & Weikart, 1993). A more recent follow-up to age 40 shows that the cost-benefit of this intervention is improving over time with the inclusion of long-term benefits (Schweinhart *et al.*, 2005). Since then (and no doubt before), the charitable sector has a strong history of publishing reports for lobbying and advocacy purposes based on the costs of *not* investing in a particular cause, such as ending child poverty (Hughes & Downie, 2000), but these have tended not to have the same strength of evidence as the Perry High/Scope work, particularly in terms of long-term follow-up.

Table 9.1 Number of times 'cost-effectiveness' comes up in searches of publications' archives for the past year.[a]

Database	Hits
British Medical Journal	162
British Journal of Social Work	4
Pulse	51
Community care	9

[a]Searches conducted on 31 July 2007.

As well as these sorts of studies of costs and resources, linking costs to outcomes (always more difficult in terms of children, where benefits and harms may take many years to appear), there has been a growing recognition of the need for an increase in studies testing cost-benefits right across the spectrum of welfare interventions beyond health.

Just as 'men are from Mars and women are from Venus' (not the most evidence-based statement in this chapter), different professions and occupations bring different strengths and skills, different histories, different approaches to leadership and different organisational cultures to the table. Within the UK, whilst education, health and social welfare are all funded from the public purse, it is undoubtedly in health that notions of cost-effectiveness have been most strongly developed and have entered professional and organisational consciousness. One way of demonstrating this is through Table 9.1, in which we looked for references to cost-effectiveness in one leading professional journal in medicine – *The British Medical Journal* and one in social care – *The British Journal of Social Work*. We then extended our searches to the more widely read (or possibly more widely received) practitioner press in medicine and in social care, again looking at one publication from each, *Community Care* for social care and *Pulse* for medicine. These were limited searches, but it can be readily seen that there are substantial differences between health and social care in terms of the exposure of readers to economic evaluations of treatment or discussion of such evaluations.

One consequence of the lack of exposure of social workers, for instance, to discussions of cost-effectiveness, is that, particularly where resources are shared, or where they are working as part of a large multidisciplinary team, they may be less well placed than their health colleagues to challenge interventions whose effectiveness and cost-effectiveness are unknown or where there is evidence of harm.

They may also, however, be at a disadvantage (and not necessarily an unfair disadvantage) as a result of the relatively scant evidence of effectiveness and cost-effectiveness in social care.

At present within the public sector in the UK, it is only in health (including both clinical interventions and public health) that economic evidence as well as evidence of effectiveness informs recommendations on treatments. As well as technical and professional expertise, NICE draws on the expertise of patients and carers, patients' organisations, nurses, doctors and other health professionals, and through its Citizens Council, a broader spectrum of opinion. The Citizens Council reports to the Board of NICE on issues ranging from whether it is appropriate when developing 'patient safety solutions' that NICE take the costs, as well as the benefits, into account, to the circumstances in which it is justified for NICE to recommend that an intervention is used only in the context of research.

Communities of Practice, effectiveness and cost-effectiveness

As we move towards more team working, more multidisciplinary working and a greater emphasis on outcomes, what part might Communities of Practice play in informing, commenting on and influencing the effectiveness and cost-effectiveness agenda?

It seems to us that the mutual engagement, joint enterprise and shared learning aspects of CoPs may well make them an important locus for promoting practice based on the best available evidence. Decision makers and practitioners are not simply people involved in the forming of pertinent questions about policies or the format for disseminating programme results. They also have the potential to become vital key informants on the mechanisms of system change. They have more access than most to both the 'supply' and the 'demand' areas of services. But even if CoPs *could* play such a role, why *should* they?

Firstly, because if they are not playing a part in informing decision makers, someone else will be. A commentator in the area of resource allocation suggests that the principal determinants of the allocation of scarce resources to improve health include the priorities of voters; the diffusion of responsibility; the absence of evidence about matters of consequence to policy-makers; the arraying of some evidence in ways that frustrate policy-making and resistance to addressing determinants other than clinical services (Fox, 2006). If he is correct, this makes it all the more important for practitioners and policy-makers with an interest in improving well-being in the widest sense – incorporating social welfare, education, justice and health – to start to garner, as well as use, evidence which might influence the allocation of scare resources.

Secondly, who better to understand the kinds of pathways between services than CoPs, which bring together professionals from different parts of the life of, for instance, a child? As Shemilt *et al.* (2008) point out, event pathways provide a systematic, explicit method of representing different criminal justice, education, social care and/or health outcomes or processes. Description of the main event pathways associated with the interventions being compared can help to clarify important items of resource use (costs) and outcomes (beneficial and adverse effects) relevant to a choice between alternative interventions. In other words, who incurs the costs, who receives the benefits and when do these costs and benefits occur. Multidisciplinary CoPs potentially have the advantage of representatives from both the sector where the money will be spent (such as early education) and the sector that may recoup the greatest financial benefit (perhaps criminal justice).

Thirdly, whilst policies may be made nationally, they are implemented (or not) locally. The cost-effectiveness of an intervention will depend on the local prevalence of the problem being addressed, how much is being done already to tackle it and what skills and resources are available locally to deal with the problem – all of which means that it is difficult to take results 'off the shelf' and apply them locally.

We do not assume that applying themselves to questions of effectiveness and cost-effectiveness will ever be the main or even a major task of a CoP – but so long as resources remain finite, it is something which needs to be kept in sight. There are, of course, problems, to which CoPs might be able to bring their own resources to bear.

At present, attempts to use the results of economic evaluations in health and social care are hampered by the paucity of data, its variable quality and its context specificity. What is more, we still do not have nearly enough really good evaluations of effectiveness of interventions or of different ways of delivering care in areas outside medicine (and not as much really sound evidence in medicine as we as patients would like to think). Communities of Practice may well be in a position when asked to implement a particular policy or practice (or thinking about their own practices) to demand the same kind of evidence of effectiveness that one might, if one were about to have a medical procedure. How likely is it to have the desired effect? What are the risks? What are the benefits? And in terms of costs, CoPs might want to consider in relation to a particular outcome what is known about the relative contribution made to a particular problem by education, health, social care or justice. Given the way that budgets are allocated, it is difficult for practitioners in different disciplines not to see themselves as in some sense in competition for the same pot of resources. Collegial work within a CoP potentially provides an opportunity to maximise holistic benefit. The benefits (and costs) of social interventions are not only *multiple* (e.g. improved health, social cohesion, employment and reduced crime), they are also *multiplied* (Shiell & Hawe, 1996). The ripples emanating from a social intervention spread wide. In economic terms we are no longer looking at changes 'at the margin', but at understanding how the fundamental properties of systems are harnessed towards socially desirable outcomes or otherwise.

In the (relative) absence of evidence, what may be needed for practitioners to make informed decisions on economically sound investments? Part of the answer lies in the 'more research is needed' which is conventionally the mantra of researchers. But part too lies in an increasing public and practitioner awareness of work on effectiveness and cost-effectiveness in service provision and development. We believe that this will depend on better practitioner/policy capacity to interpret, translate, apply (and where necessary, challenge) economic evidence locally. It is probably at a local level too that professionals will be best placed to consider what will *not* be done in order to accommodate new investments and interventions (the economic notion of opportunity cost). Communities of Practice, where practitioners and professionals are well placed to comment on both costs and effectiveness, to question data, and to have an awareness (along with users) of the most important outcomes to measure, may well have a crucial part to play in this.

In health care since the early 1990s, the Cochrane Collaboration has played a key role in assembling research evidence on effectiveness. The Campbell Collaboration is now starting to do the same in education, social welfare and criminal justice. Shemilt *et al.* (2008), who are working on ways of looking at cost-effectiveness, suggest a number of questions – some of which might be considered by a CoP in a particular substantive area, or in relation to a population group:

- What is the economic burden placed on society (e.g. individuals, groups and service providers) by the social problem(s) which the alternative courses of action under consideration (i.e. intervention and comparators) are seeking to address?
- What types of resource inputs/costs (e.g. staff, equipment and premises) are likely to be required in order to implement and sustain the alternative courses of action under consideration?
- What are the potential resource consequences of implementing the alternative courses of action under consideration? *Or* how might the alternative courses of action under consideration impact on the subsequent use of resources?
- What is the economic value associated with changes in outcomes that may result from one course of action compared with another (i.e. intervention vs comparators)?
- Who bears the costs (resource inputs, resource consequences), who receives the benefits and when do costs and benefits occur?
- What are the potential trade-offs between costs (resource use) and beneficial or adverse effects that may need to be considered in a decision to adopt or reject a given course of action?

For funding to be directed towards effective and away from ineffective or harmful interventions involves having the data and knowledge to make informed choices. Access to these data and knowledge, however, is not only needed by the economists who can do the specialist work needed on cost-benefit analyses. The knowledge, and the opportunity to influence the ways in which this knowledge is framed, collected and valued is an issue for practitioners in the areas where we want to know what the most cost-effective interventions are. Those in CoP may well have close links with users of services, and local communities, with specialist expertise to contribute on the kinds of outcomes which they value. This suggests that practitioners (as well as users and citizens) need to be engaged in the creation of economic evidence from the very beginning.

Finally, and perhaps more controversially, CoPs are themselves interventions since they are a use of a scarce resource which might be used for some other purpose. One good way of understanding effectiveness and cost-effectiveness would be to construct a simple model of desired outcomes and set these against resources expended. Not everything 'works' and not everything 'works' straightaway, but this kind of evaluation can be worthwhile. If it is not working, there are plenty of other useful demands on time.

Chapter 10

WHERE DOES THIS GET US AND WHERE WILL WE GO FROM HERE?

Andrée le May

This book has shown that despite their sometimes unpredictable and complex nature, Communities of Practice (CoPs) can positively impact on:

- the standard of care delivered to patients/clients;
- the working environments and job satisfaction of the participants in the community;
- the ways in which people exchange knowledge and learn;
- the ways in which problems are solved;
- the speed with which knowledge and innovation move into practice;
- the generation of knowledge from practice;
- the creation of a unified team which may be uni- or multi-professional; and
- the ownership and sustainability of changes to practice.

We have also seen how successful CoPs can increase social, human, organisational, professional and patient/client capital even if, in some instances, uncertainties about and dislike of the CoP label and its associated jargon stand in the way of their introduction, development and progress.

Recently, there has been increased interest in 'researching' CoPs, watching and asking about how knowledge is shared, how learning occurs and how this learning impacts on the development of professional practice. Whilst we need to continue to be inquisitive about the impact that CoPs have on learning and knowledge transfer, we also need to map and compare the different ways in which CoPs are constructed and function, be they face-to-face or virtual, and how they compare with other more conventional approaches to learning.

In addition to this general extension of our knowledge of CoPs, those of us working and researching in health and social care need to know and articulate their worth in our arena. Undoubtedly, there are plenty of observations and stories of CoPs in health and social care, some of which you have read in the chapters of this book that help us to understand what goes on in them and between them and their host organisations. However, these mainly qualitative data alone do not give us enough information about the effectiveness, let alone the cost-effectiveness of the CoPs when compared to other techniques for learning and changing practice. They tell us about worth in terms of experiences, of the transfer of knowledge, of learning and of people's preferences for learning, but when you are confronted with hard choices about how to spend money in health and social care, these data are insufficient. We need to complement them with more quantifiable evidence so that we can stretch our understanding from simply knowing how and why CoPs work to knowing if they are the most efficient and cost-effective way to develop learning and change practice in various health and social care settings. If CoPs really are to become an enduring feature of health and social care practices and not just an early twenty-first-century vogue, we need to know if they are the right option to choose intellectually, practically, economically and socially.

Whilst finding out more about CoPs' effectiveness is one of the key areas for development in the future, it is also important to focus on how CoPs develop professional and patient/client capital and integrate these into practice. We need to find answers to many questions if we are to continue to take advantage of this facet of learning in CoPs. For instance, how is knowledge built in CoPs between experts – be they professionals or patients/clients and novices? How do CoPs shape the sociocultural practices of a profession or a patient/client group? How do CoPs clustered around patients/clients interact and transfer knowledge and learning to those built around professionals and vice versa? What are the main components of professional and patient/client capital, and how do CoPs link with other structures, formal and informal, to generate and enhance them?

In addition to this – and assuming that the evaluations of CoPs' effectiveness prove favourable – we need to consider how trust, willingness to share knowledge and the social infrastructures that foster learning in CoPs can be further developed and inculcated into virtual communities, which may or may not be associated with face-to-face interaction. The infusion of social networking websites into our lives during the last 5 years leaves the door open for combining this technology with some of the ideas that underpin CoPs. If it is possible to merge these two concepts, then we could experience the benefits linked to CoPs more widely across health and social care. In North America there are already subscription-only websites (e.g. www.within3.com and www.sermo.com) targeted at doctors and other health care workers, which enable them to ask questions of each other, use the answers to alter their practice and then feed back on the usefulness of the answers. A new site in the UK takes this a step closer to the concept of the CoP by clustering the virtual social networks around specific geographical locations, specialist practice and groups of practitioners already known to each other. This site – www.KaseBook.net – is being piloted with doctors and nurses working in primary care and if successful promises to revolutionise the way clinicians learn from each other.

Although the success of these initiatives has not been evaluated, they do appear to have the potential to combine some of the more positive features of CoPs including the willingness to share knowledge and the ability, over time, to build trust between participants, which in turn develops the social infrastructures that foster learning. Indeed it might be possible, once they have matured, to establish if they hold the components of the social theory of learning – meaning, practice, community and identity that Wenger described (1998: 5). As you remember from Chapter 1, he defined each of these components as follows:

'*Meaning*: a way of talking about our (changing) ability – individually and collectively – to experience our life and the world as meaningful' (in terms of learning, he refers to this as 'learning as experience').

'*Practice*: a way of talking about shared historical and social resources, frameworks and perspectives that can sustain mutual engagement in action' (in terms of learning, he refers to this as 'learning as doing').

'*Community*: a way of talking about the social configurations in which our enterprises are defined as worth pursuing and our participation is recognizable as competence' (in terms of learning, he refers to this as 'learning as belonging').

'*Identity*: a way of talking about how learning changes who we are and creates personal histories of becoming in the context of our communities' (in terms of learning, he refers to this as 'learning as becoming').

Whilst 'talking' in the literal sense is not possible on these social networking, websites, better web cams and video-conferencing techniques will mean that 'virtual' face-to-face interactions are not too far away. If these innovations encourage the successful development of CoPs, more and more health and social care practitioners and patients/clients will find themselves interacting, learning and sharing knowledge in CoPs, and as a result of this easier transfer of knowledge, best practice will be shared, professional and patient/client capital increased and care should improve. After all, it is the desire to improve one's practical knowledge, and not the method of communication, that drives a CoP.

These social networking websites are seductive developments, melding the key characteristics of CoPs with highly sophisticated technology, thereby making them highly accessible, easy to use and as such a potentially quick route to CoP development and maintenance and, through the CoPs, to the enhancement of professional capital. However, focusing too strongly on social networking technologies may make us lose sight of the varied application of the CoP concept that has led to its current popularity. It is important not to abandon the old for the new, but rather to find ways of sustaining both.

Successful learning in CoPs, whether face-to-face or virtual, deliberately established, naturally emerging, or fostered through a social networking website, will need to take account of the essence of the CoP – that it enables learning and knowledge to evolve through the social process of interacting with like-minded people. Nurturing this essence is likely to keep the concept healthy well into the future.

REFERENCES

Agar, M. (1996) *The Professional Stranger*. Academic Press, San Diego.

Alani, H., O'Hara, K. & Shadbolt, N. (2002) ONTOCOPI: methods and tools for identifying communities of practice. In: *Proceedings of the 17th IFIP World Computer Congress*, Montreal, Canada.

Arai, L., Popay, J., Roen, K. & Roberts, H. (2005) It might work in Oklahoma but will it work in Oakhampton? What does the effectiveness literature on domestic smoke detectors tell us about context and implementation? *Injury Prevention*, 11, 148–51.

Ardichvili, A., Page, V. & Wentling, T. (2003) Motivation and barriers to participation in virtual knowledge-sharing communities of practice. *Journal of Knowledge Management*, 7 (1), 64–77.

Barnardo's Research and Development (2000) *What Works?: Making Connections: Linking Research and Practice*. Barnardo's, Ilford.

Barnett, W. S. (1993) Cost benefit analysis. In: *The High/Scope Perry Preschool Study Through Age 27* (eds L. J. Schweinhart, H. V. Barnes & D. P. Weikart). High/Scope Educational Research Foundation, Ypsilanti.

Bate, P. (2004) The role of stories and storytelling in organizational change efforts: the anthropology of an intervention within a UK hospital. *Intervention Research*, 1 (1), 27–42.

Bate, P. & Robert, G. (2002) Knowledge management and communities of practice in the private sector: lessons for modernizing the National Health Service in England and Wales. *Public Administration*, 80 (4), 643–63.

Becker, A. L. (1991) A short essay on languaging. In: *Research and Reflexivity* (ed. F. Steier). Sage, London.

Becker, G. (1964, 1993) *Human Capital: A Theoretical and Empirical Analysis, with Special Reference to Education*, 3rd edn. University of Chicago Press, Chicago.

Berg, M. & Mol, A. (1998) *Differences in Medicine: Unraveling Practices, Techniques, and Bodies*. Duke University Press, Durham and London.

Berman, P. A., Gwatkin, D. R. & Burger, S. E. (1987) Community-based health workers: head start or false start towards health for all? *Social Science and Medicine*, 25 (5), 443–59.

Billett, S. (2002) Critiquing workplace learning discourses: participation and continuity at work. *Studies in the Education of Adults*, 34 (1), 56–67.

Black, S. & Lynch, L. (2005) Measuring organizational capital in the new economy. In: *Measuring Capital in the New Economy* (eds C. Corrado, J. Haltiwanger & D. Sichel). National Bureau of Economic Research Studies in Income and Wealth. The University of Chicago Press, Chicago.

Blaxter, M. (1983) The causes of disease. Women talking. *Social Science and Medicine*, 17 (2), 59–69.

Boud, D. & Middleton, H. (2003) Learning from others at work: communities of practice and informal learning. *Journal of Workplace Learning*, 15 (5), 194–202.

Boud, D., Cohen, R. & Walker, D. (1993) *Using Experience for Learning*. SRHE and Open University Press, Buckingham.

Bourdieu, P. (1990) *The Logic of Practice*. Polity Press, London.

Bradshaw, A. (1994) *Lighting the Lamp: The Spiritual Dimension of Nursing Care*. Scutari, London.

Brocklehurst, N. & Liabo, K. (2004) Evidence nuggets: promoting evidence-based practice. *Community Practitioner*, 77 (10), 292–6.

Brown, J. S. & Duguid, P. (1991) Organizational learning and communities-of-practice: toward a unified view of working, learning and innovation. *Organization Science*, 2 (1), 40–57.

Brown, J. S. & Duguid, P. (2000) *The Social Life of Information*. Harvard Business School Press, Harvard.

Brown, J. S. & Duguid, P. (2001) Knowledge and organization. *Organization Science*, 12 (2), 198–213.

Bryant-Lukosius, D. & DiCenso, A. (2004) A framework for the introduction and evaluation of advanced practice nursing roles. *Journal of Advanced Nursing*, 48 (5), 530–40.

Cabinet Office (1998) *Better Government for Older People Programme (BGOP)*. Cabinet Office, London.

Callon, M. (1986) Some elements of a sociology of translation: domestication of the scallops and the fishermen of St Brieuc Bay. In: *Power, Action and Belief: A new sociology of knowledge?* (ed. J. Law). Routledge and Kegan Paul, London.

Calnan, M. (1987) *Health and Illness*. Tavistock, London.

Carroll, L. (1929) *Alice's Adventures in Wonderland. Through the Looking Class and Other Works*. Marshall Cavendish Partworks Ltd [1987 edition], London.

Cayton, H. (2004) Foreword. In: *Patient and Public Involvement in Health: The Evidence for Policy Implementation*. Department of Health, London.

Chau, C. (2005) Professional capital: an informational approach to nursing. In: *Proceedings of the 2005 International Conference on Knowledge Management*, North Carolina.

Chiou, C., Hay, J., Wallace, J. F. Bloom, B., Neumann, P., Sullivan, S., Yu, H., Keeler, E., Henning, J. & Ofman, J. (2003) Development and validation of a grading system for the quality of cost-effectiveness studies. *Medical Care*, 41 (1), 32–44.

CHSRF (2003a) *Final Report from the Executive Training for Research Application Proposed Program Design and Development, Final Report of the Design Working Group*. Available at: www.chsrf.ca/extra/pdf/Final_Planning_Report_e.pdf (accessed 17 October 2003).

CHSRF (2003b) *Strategic Plan 2003–2007*. CHSRF, Ottawa.

CHSRF (2007) *Executive Training for Research Application 2007 Guide for Applicants*. Available at: http://www.chsrf.ca/extra/pdf/2007_EXTRA guide_e.pdf (accessed 31 July 2007).

CHSRF, CAN, CCHSE, le Consortium quebecios & CMA (2004) Memorandum of Agreement. CHSRF, Canada.

Coakes, E. & Smith, P. (2006) *Using Communities of Practice for Sustainable Change Management*. Paper presented at Knowledge Management Aston Conference. Birmingham, UK.

Coulter, A. (2006) *Engaging Patients in Their Healthcare*. Picker Institute Europe, Oxford.

Cox, A. (2005) What are communities of practice? A comparative review of four seminal works. *Journal of Information Science*, 31 (6), 527–40.

Crisp, N. (2007) *Global Health Partnerships: The UK Contribution to Health in Developing Countries.* Department of Health, London.

Czarniawska, B. (1997) *Narrating the Organization.* University of Chicago Press, Chicago.

Daniel, B., Schwier, R. & McCalla, G. (2003) Social capital in virtual leaning communities and distributed communities of practice. *Canadian Journal of Learning and Technology,* 29 (3), 113–39.

Daniel, J. (1998) *Knowledge Media for Mega-Universities: Scaling Up New Technology at The Open University.* Shanghai Open and Distance Learning Symposium. Available at: www.open.ac.uk/johndanielspeeches/chinatlk.htm (accessed 31 July 2007).

Davenport, T. & Prusak, L. (1998) *Working Knowledge: How Organisations Manage What They Know.* Harvard Business School Press, Harvard.

Denning, S. (2005a) Using narrative as a tool for change. In: *Storytelling in Organizations* (eds J. Seely Brown, S. Denning, K. Groh & L. Prusak). Elsevier Butterworth-Heinemann, Burlington.

Denning, S. (2005b) The role of narrative in organizations. In: *Storytelling in Organizations* (eds J. Seely Brown, S. Denning, K. Groh & L. Prusak). Elsevier Butterworth-Heinemann, Burlington.

Department of Health (2000) *The NHS Plan.* The Stationery Office Limited, London.

Department of Health (2001) *National Service Framework for Older People.* Department of Health, London.

Department of Health (2002) *The Expert Patient: A New Approach to Chronic Disease Management for the 21st Century.* Department of Health, London.

Department of Health (2004) *Trust Me I'm a Patient: A Patient and Public Involvement Game.* Department of Health, London.

Department of Health (2005a) *The National Service Framework for Renal Services Part Two: Chronic Kidney Disease, Acute Renal Failure and End of Life Care.* Department of Health, London.

Department of Health (2005b) *About Our health, Our Care, Our Say.* Available at: www.dh.gov.uk/PolicyAndGuidance/OrganisationPolicy/Modernisation (accessed 16 August 2007).

Department of Health (2006a) *Revisions to the GMS Contract 2006/7: Delivering Investment in General Practice.* Department of Health, London.

Department of Health (2006b) *A Stronger Local Voice: A Framework for Creating a Stronger Local Voice in the Development of Health and Social Care Services.* Department of Health, London.

DIPEx Available at: http://www.dipex.org/ (accessed 16 August 2007).

Du Bois, D. L., Holloway, B. E., Valentine, J. C. & Cooper, H. (2002) Effectiveness of mentoring programs for youth: a meta-analytic review. *American Journal of Community Psychology,* 30 (2), 157–97.

Edwards, D. & Potter, J. (1992) *Discursive Psychology.* Sage, London.

Eriksen, T. (2001) *Small Places, Large Issues: An Introduction to Social and Cultural Anthropology.* Pluto Press, London.

Evenson, R. & Westphal, L. (1995) Technological change and technology strategy. In: *Handbook of Development Economics* (eds J. Behrman & T. N. Srinivasan). 3A, Amsterdam.

Exley, B. (2001) Teachers' professional knowledge: tensions within the accounts of off shore instruction. In: *Designing Educational Research: Theories, Methods and Practices* (eds P. Singh & E. McWilliam). Post Pressed, Flaxton.

Foucault, M. (1972) *The Archaeology of Knowledge* [translated by A. M. Sheridan Smith]. Routledge, London.

Foucault, M. (1973) *The Birth of the Clinician – Archaeology of Medical Perception* [translated by A. M. Sheridan Smith]. Routledge, London.

Fountain, D. & Arbreton, A. (1999) The cost of mentoring. In: *Contemporary Issues in Mentoring* (ed. J. B. Grossman). Public Private Ventures, Philadelphia.

Fox, S. (2000) Communities of practice, Foucault and actor-network theory. *Journal of Management Studies*, 37 (6), 853–67.

Frost, S., Moseley, A., Tierney, S., Ellis, A., Duffy, M., Hutton, A. & Newman, T. (2005) *The Evidence Guide: Using Research and Evaluation in Social Care and Allied Professions.* Barnardo's, Barkingside.

Gabbay, J. & le May, A. (2004) Evidence-based guidelines or collectively constructed 'mindlines'? Ethnographic study of knowledge management in primary care. *British Medical Journal*, 329, 1013–17.

Gabbay, J., le May, A., Jefferson, H., Webb, D., Lovelock, R. Powell, J. & Lathlean, J. (2003) A case study of knowledge management in multi-agency consumer-informed 'communities of practice': implications for evidence-based policy development in health and social services. *Health: An Interdisciplinary Journal for the Social Study of Health, Illness and Medicine*, 7 (3), 283–310.

Gadamer, H. G. (1973) Concerning empty and full-filled time. In: *Martin Heidegger in Europe and America* (eds E. G. Ballard & C. E. Scott). Martinus Nijhoff, The Hague.

Gadamer, H. G. (1993) *Truth and Method* [translation J. Weinsheimer & D. G. Marshall]. Second revised edition of the 1975 original Sheed and Ward, London.

Gibson, F. (2006) *Reminiscence and Recall.* Age Concern, London.

Gobbi, M. (2005) Nursing practice as bricoleur activity: a concept explored. *Nursing Inquiry*, 12 (2), 117–25.

Goldenberg, M. J. (2005) Evidence-based ethics? On evidence-based practice and the 'empirical turn' from normative bioethics. *BMC Medical Ethics*, 6 (11), 2621–2632.

Goode, W. J. (1957) Community within a community: the professions. *American Sociological Review*, 22 (2), 194–200.

Goodwin, C. (1994) Professional vision. *American Anthropologist*, 96 (3), 606–33.

Gray, J. A. M. (2001) *Evidence-Based Healthcare. How to Make Health Policy and Management Decisions.* Churchill Livingstone, Edinburgh.

Greenhalgh, T. (1999) Narrative-based medicine in an evidence-based world. *British Medical Journal*, 318 (7179), 323–5.

Grossman, J. B. & Tierney, J. P. (1998) Does mentoring work? An impact study of the Big Brothers Big Sisters program, *Evaluation Review*, 22 (3), 403–26.

Haines, A. & Donald, A. (1998) *Getting Research into Practice.* BMJ Books, London.

Hamric, A. B. (2005) Role development of the advanced practice nurse. In: *Advanced Practice Nursing: An Integrative Approach* (eds A. B. Hamric, J. A. Spross & C. M. Hanson). Elsevier Saunders, St. Louis.

Hanks, W. (1991) Foreword. In: *Situated Learning: Legitimate Peripheral Participation* (eds J. Lave & E. Wenger). Cambridge University Press, Cambridge and New York.

Havens, K. K., Wagstaff, D. A., Mercer, P. A., Longeway, K. & Gutman, M. (1997) Lessons learned from a mentoring program for teenage mothers. *Wisconsin Medical Journal*, 96 (9), 38–43.

Health Canada and CHSRF (2003) *Funding Agreement between Health Canada and CHSRF.* CHSRF, Canada.

Hepworth, M. (2000) *Stories of Ageing.* Open University Press, Buckingham.

Herzlich, C. (1973) *Health and Illness*. Graham, H. (Tr), Academic Press, London.

Hughes, M. & Downie, A. S. N. (2000) *Counting the Cost of Child Poverty*, Barnardo's, Barkingside.

Iyigun, M. F. & Owen, A. L. (1999) Entrepreneurs, professionals and growth. *Journal of Economic Growth*, 4, 213–32.

Jerrome, D. (1992) *Good Company: An Anthropological Study of Old People in Groups.* Edinburgh University Press, Edinburgh.

Johnson, C. M. (2001) A survey of current research on online communities. *The Internet and Higher Education*, 4 (1), 45–60.

Kirkpatrick, F. G. (1991) Introduction. In: *Persons in Relation*, Vol. 2 (ed. J. Macmurray) of The Form of the Personal. [Re-issue of the 1961 edition with a new introduction by Frank G. Kirkpatrick, 1991]. Humanities Press International. New Jersey.

Knowles, M. S., Holton, E. F., III & Swanson, R. A. (2005) *The Adult Learner*, 6th edn. Elsevier Butterworth-Heinmann, London.

Lathlean, J. & le May, A. (2002) Communities of practice: an opportunity for interagency working. *Journal of Clinical Nursing*, 11 (3), 394–8.

Latour, B. (1987) *Science in Action: How to Follow Scientists and Engineers Through Society.* Open University Press, Buckingham.

Lave, J. & Wenger, E. (1991) *Situated Learning: Legitimate Peripheral Participation.* Cambridge University Press, Cambridge and New York.

Leahey, E. (2006) *Specialisation and Integration in Publication and Patenting Activity.* Paper presented at the NSF sponsored workshop using Human Resource data from SRS to Study the S & E Workforce.

le May, A. (1998) Empowering older people through communication. In: *Health and Empowerment: Research and Practice* (ed. S. Kendall). Edward Arnold, London.

Lesser, E. & Prusak, L. (1999) *Communities of Practice, Social Capital and Organizational Knowledge.* Institute of Knowledge Management, Cambridge, MA.

Lesser, E. & Storck, J. (2001) Communities of practice and organizational performance. *IBM Systems Journal*, 40 (4), 831–41.

Llewellyn, N. (2001) The role of storytelling and narrative in a modernisation initiative. *Local Government Studies*, 27 (4), 35–58.

Lomas, J. (2000) Using 'linkage and exchange' to move research into policy at a Canadian Foundation. *Health Affairs*, 19, 236–40.

Macmurray, J. (1961) *Persons in Relation*, Vol. 2 of The Form of the Personal. [Re-issue of the 1961 edition with a new introduction by Frank.G. Kirkpatrick, 1991]. Humanities Press International, New Jersey.

Malikail, J. (2003) Moral character: Hexis, Habitus and 'Habit'. *An Internet Journal of Philosophy*, 7, 1–22.

McGregor, S. (2004) *Philosophical Well-being*. Working Paper. Available at: http://www.kon.org/hswp/archive/philosophical.pdf (accessed 5 December 2007).

Mol, A. M. (2002) *The Body Multiple: Ontology in Medical Practice.* Duke University Press, Durham and London.

Nahapiet, J. & Ghoshal, S. (1998) Social capital, intellectual capital, and the organizational advantage. *The Academy of Management Review*, 23 (2), 242–66.

NHS Executive Northern and Yorkshire (1999) *Public Engagement Toolkit for Primary Care Groups.* NHS Executive Northern and Yorkshire.

Nonaka, I. & Takeuchi, H. (1995) *The Knowledge Creating Company: How Japanese Companies Create the Dynamics of Innovation.* Oxford University Press, Oxford.

Polanyi, M. (1958) *Personal Knowledge*. Routledge and Kegan Paul, London.

Polanyi, M. (1983) *The Tacit Dimension*. Peter Smith, Gloucester, MA.

Polanyi, M. (1985) Conversational storytelling. Discourse and dialogue. In: *Handbook of Discourse Analysis* (ed. T. van Dijk). Academic Press, London.

Putnam, R. (2000) *Bowling Alone: The Collapse and Revival of American Community*. New York, Simon & Schuster, London.

Ramaswamy, R., Storer, G. & van Zeyl, R. (2005) Designing sustainable communities at CARE. *Knowledge Management for Development Journal*, 1 (1) 79–93.

Schweinhart, L. J. & Weikart, D. P. (1993) *A Summary of Significant Benefits: The High/Scope Perry Pre-School Study Through Age 27*. High/Scope Press, Ypsilanti.

Schweinhart, L. J., Montie, J., Xiang, Z., Barnett, W. S. & Nores, M. (2005) *Lifetime Effects: The High/Scope Perry Preschool Study Through Age 40*. High/Scope Press, Ypsilanti.

Sculpher, M., Pang, F., Manca, A., Drummond, M.F., Golder, S., Urdahl, H., Davies, L.M. & Eastwood, A. (2004) *Generalisability in Economic Evaluation Studies in Healthcare: A Review and Case Studies*. Health Technology Assessment, 8.

Seely Brown, J. (2005) Narrative as a knowledge medium in organizations. In: *Storytelling in Organizations* (eds J. Seely Brown, S. Denning, K. Groh & L. Prusak). Elsevier Butterworth-Heinemann, Burlington.

Seely Brown, J., Denning, S., Groh, K. & Prusak, L. (2005) *Storytelling in Organizations*. Elsevier Butterworth-Heinemann, Burlington.

Sergiovanni, T. J. (1998) Leadership as pedagogy, capital development and school effectiveness. *International Journal of Leadership in Education*, 1 (1), 37–46.

Shemilt, I., Mugford, M., Byford, S., Drummond, M., Eisenstein, E., Knapp, M., Mallender, J., Marsh, K., McDaid, M., Vale, L. & Walker, D. (2008) *The Campbell Collaboration Economics Methods Policy Brief*, C2 Methods Group.

Shiell, A. & Hawe, P. (1996) Health promotion, community development and the tyranny of individualism. *Health Economics*, 5, 241–7.

Shorter Oxford Dictionary (1973) Vol. II. Oxford University Press.

Shotter, J. (1975) *Images of Man in Psychological Research*. Methuen and Co. Ltd, London.

Shotter, J. (1993) *Conversational Realities: Constructing Life through Language*. Sage, London.

Spradley, J. (1979) *The Ethnographic Interview*. Harcourt Brace Jovanovich Inc., Florida.

Stacey, M. (1994) The power of lay knowledge. In: *Researching the People's Health* (eds J. Poppay & G. Williams). Routledge, London.

Steier, F. (1991) *Research and Reflexivity*. Sage, London.

Stevens, M., Liabo, K., Frost, S. & Roberts, H. (2005) Using research in practice. A research information service for social care practitioners. *Child and Family Social Work*, 10 (1), 67–75.

Stevens, M., Liabo, K. & Roberts, H. (2007) A review of the research priorities of practitioners working with children in social care. *Child and Family Social Work*, 12 (4), 295–305.

Stevens, M., Shiell, A. & Roberts, H. (2008) *What Works, What Matters and What Counts: Preliminary Work on Cost Effectiveness in Social Care with Children*. Report for the Nuffield Foundation.

St James-Roberts, I. & Samlal Singh, C. (2001) *Can Mentors Help Primary School Children with Behaviour Problems? Final Report of the Thomas Coram Research Unit between March 1997 and 2000*. Home Office Research, Development and Statistics Directorate, 233.

Tarling, R., Burrows, J. & Clarke, A. (2001) *Dalston Youth Projects Part II (11-14): An evaluation*. Home Office Research, Development and Statistics Directorate, 232.

Thompson, M. (2005) Structural and epistemic parameters in communities of practice. *Organization Science*, 16 (2), 151–64.

Tierney, J. P., Grossman, J. B. & Resch, N. L. (2000) *Making a difference. An impact study of Big Brothers Big Sisters*. Public Private Ventures, Philadelphia.

Trinder, L. & Reynolds, S. (2000) *Evidence-Based Practice: A critical appraisal*. Blackwell Science. Oxford.

Usher, R. (1992) Experience in adult education: a post-modern critique. *Journal of Philosophy of Education*, 1 (2), 201–14.

van Winkelen, C. (2003) *Inter-organisational Communities of Practice*. Working Paper, Henley Management College.

Warner, M. (1994) *Managing Monsters: Six Myths of Our Time*. Vintage, London.

Weick, K. (1995) *Sensemaking in Organizations*. Sage Publications. Thousand Oaks.

Weick, K. (2001) *Making Sense of the Organization*. Blackwell Publishing Ltd. Oxford, UK and Malden, MA.

Wenger, E. (1996) Communities of practice. The social fabric of a learning organization. *Healthcare Forum Journal*, July–August, 20–26.

Wenger, E. (1998) *Communities of Practice: Learning, Meaning and Identity*. Cambridge University Press. New York.

Wenger, E. (2006) EXTRA workshop. CHSRF, Canada.

Wenger, E. (2007) EXTRA workshop. CHSRF, Canada.

Wenger, E., McDermott, R. & Snyder, W. (2002) *Cultivating Communities of Practice*. Harvard Business School, Harvard.

Williams, R. (1990) *A Protestant Legacy: Attitudes to Death and Illness Among Older Aberdonians*. Clarendon Press, Oxford.

World Health Organisation (1987) *Community Health Workers, Working Document SHS/HMD/SG.87.4*. WHO, Geneva.

World Health Organisation (2004a) *World Health Report – Changing History*. WHO, Geneva.

World Health Organisation (2004b) *World Health Statistics*. WHO, Geneva.

World Health Organisation (2006) *World Health Report – Working Together for Health*. WHO, Geneva.

Zadeh, L. & Yager, R. (1987) Fuzzy Sets and Applications. Wiley, New York.

INDEX